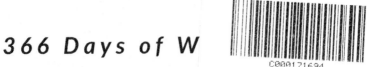

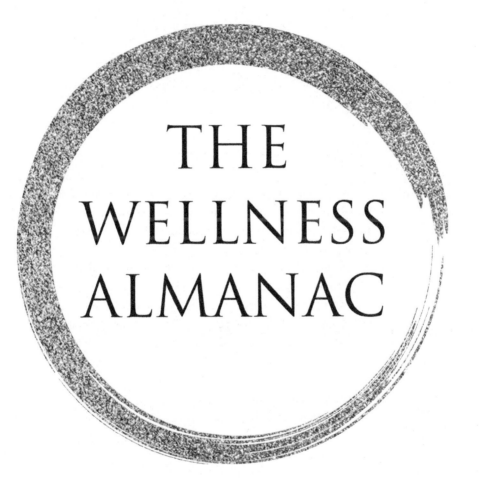

THE
WELLNESS
ALMANAC

ISABEL CARTER

Cover image by: Alex_82, 99Designs
Editing and proofreading by: Craig Smith (CRS Editorial)
Book design by: SWATT Books Ltd

Printed in the United Kingdom
First Printed 2023

ISBN: 978-1-7394339-0-1 (Paperback)
ISBN: 978-1-7394339-1-8 (eBook)

Isabel Carter
Heckmondwike, West Yorkshire WF16 9AA

www.yogainsideout.co.uk

Contents

---

366 Days of Wellbeing

Introduction

Welcome to *The Wellness Almanac* and to what I hope will be 366 days of wellbeing! Thank you for joining me. Please thank yourself for having the wisdom to open this book.

This book has been in my mind for many years. As a copious and diligent collector of all things wellbeing, I was inspired to collate my wisdom during the Covid-19 lockdowns. I have always felt it important to share what I learn, so I decided that one way I could help my yoga students and Facebook followers was by posting a wellbeing tip every day we were locked down – sharing the things I was doing myself to stay well during this time. These tips went down very well. I received many messages of thanks and, more importantly, messages telling me how much the tips were helping people. It was this feedback that provided the push I needed.

Some of you will be interested to read my story and the reasons behind the principles that guide me – I hope I offer some light. I recognise others will want to dive right into the book – you have no need to know me! Therefore, please feel free to skip ahead, should you wish. Indeed, skip any pages that don't thrill you – this isn't a school textbook! Let it unfold in whatever way works best for you.

For over 30 years I have been practising yoga in various forms, though didn't experience the feeling of having "come home" until I found Dru Yoga, shortly after the passing of my much-loved dad. I consider myself blessed to have discovered Dru Yoga's potential for healing at a young age. It certainly helped me navigate my way through a difficult time and has been my constant friend since. I welcome the connection to the natural world and the energy of the seasons, which this ancient philosophy inspires. It is a source of ongoing joy, not to mention healing – never more so than when I was diagnosed with a serious and challenging autoimmune condition in 2016. As always, I turned to my beloved yoga practices and the wisdom that presents itself whenever I need it. Without going into detail (that's for another time!), I healed myself so quickly that my consultant at the hospital was surprised and reluctant to discharge me at first as he couldn't believe what he was seeing! A big part of my healing process alongside yoga was delving deeper into Ayurveda, the system for maintaining good health. This reinforced my relationship with the seasons and the elements, building on my existing knowledge of how to harness and balance the energy of both to support health and wellbeing.

I am pleased to say I haven't had any recurrence of my autoimmune disease, and the irritating little ones I always thought were just part of life, such as hay fever and migraines, have also disappeared. Every time I put these practices to the test (and I really do test them, as I'm a sceptic by nature!), they work. I'm very much a practical person. If something doesn't work, I can't see the point of doing it, so you can be assured the wisdom I share is practical **and** effective.

As I move into the next phase of my life – and all the fun things that come with the menopause – my yoga and associated practices continue to keep my mind, body and emotions balanced; healthy and harmonious. My greatest wish is that, as you navigate your world, this book becomes a wise friend, encouraging and inspiring you to take good care of yourself...and I hope you enjoy it too!

How to Get the Most From This Book

As already alluded to, it was always my heartfelt intention for this book to become a trusted companion – a source of practical wisdom packed with simple, effective techniques to help us move smoothly through our busy world. The last thing I want is for it to become in any way onerous, or to feel like another chore to add to your list. It's certainly not a failure if you don't read and implement every idea. When it comes to getting the most out of this book, there are no rules. It really is your choice.

Maybe you are ready to start 1 January, eager to explore a year of wellness. It's just as easy though to start on any day that suits you. Each tip stands alone, with many being season-specific. Therefore, when you start isn't important...just start. You may prefer a less structured approach, dipping in and out as the mood takes you, which works just as well.

I sincerely hope you become inspired to use the book for many years. There is always something new to discover. Tips that didn't speak to you last year maybe just what you need to hear this year and, oh, the joy of rediscovering a little gem of wisdom that served you well but you'd since forgotten about!

By the side of each day you will see a symbol denoting the area of wellbeing the tip benefits - many of the tips are multipurpose! This way, you can swiftly locate the information you need, without having to read through the whole book. The categories are as follows:

 Calm, clarity and relaxation
 Digestive support

Energy boost

☆ Graceful ageing

 Moving with ease

 Seasonal

Zzz Sleep

♡ Wellness.

I've been tapping into the wisdom of the seasons for many years, filling many notebooks with all manner of information. Here are a few pointers that have helped me along the way and that I hope help you too:

- Delve into the book with an open mind. You don't have to like or find every tip useful, or even try everything. Simply be a curious excavator of the wellbeing gems that work for you.
- Give the tips and techniques a fair chance. Just reading about them or trying them once is unlikely to yield great results.
- Never tolerate pain or discomfort. If something doesn't feel right in any way, then stop. Listen to your body. Seek advice from your healthcare provider if you are in doubt or concerned.
- The wisdom shared is intended as a complementary practice to support your wellbeing. The information is not intended as a replacement for whatever medical treatment you might be undergoing or to replace the advice of your healthcare provider.
- Most important of all...enjoy yourself.

A little bit more on the health considerations

The Wellness Almanac is all about taking the best care of ourselves and honouring our bodies, each and every day of the year. This means listening to our bodies, taking the advice of our healthcare practitioners, and missing out or modifying any of the tips and techniques that do not work for you. If you have any underlying health concerns, please consult with your healthcare provider before starting.

Most of the tips are safe for everyone. Where appropriate, I have highlighted health considerations or where extra care is required. Never tolerate pain or discomfort. **If anything hurts, feels uncomfortable on any level, or you just don't like it, then STOP! Speak to an appropriate healthcare professional before you continue.** Pain and discomfort are some of the ways our body communicates with us. Listen to this inner wisdom, reassess and seek advice.

This book is not suitable if you are prenatal or postnatal. At this time, you need special nurturing, with practices dedicated to you and your baby.

Foundation Principles

Some of the ideas and tips I present might be new to you, which is why I have included a short section on the fundamental principles of holistic wellbeing.

It's not necessary to read this section to enjoy or benefit from the ideas presented in the book. You may already be knowledgeable, or eager to dive straight in, in which case please do! Just remember that you can always refer to these principles, should you need to.

Ayurveda

Ayurveda is often described as the sister science of yoga, offering a natural and holistic system for good health. The word "Ayurveda" comes from the Sanskrit words "ayur" (meaning "life") and "veda" (which is translated as "science" or "knowledge"). Put simply, it works on the basic principle that everything in life is made up of three doshas (see page 12) in different proportions. When these proportions become out of balance, disease can set in. Ayurveda uses a variety of methods such as dietary advice, lifestyle tweaks, herbal remedies, movement and gemstones, primarily to maintain good health and restore harmony if disease sets in.

If you are interested in Ayurveda and have a condition you would like help with, I urge you to seek the advice of a qualified practitioner. There is a lot of information out there, but we are individuals and one size does not fit all, so the chances of finding the exact "prescription" for you is minimal. We can, though, employ some of the basic Ayurvedic wellness principles to help us maintain our equilibrium and good health, and even ease mild symptoms of many common ailments.

It is a truly holistic healthcare system that considers the uniqueness of every one of us.

The Five Elements

This book looks at the five elements – earth, water, fire, air and space (also known as ether) – that are present in our natural environment, and that we can connect with as we move through the seasons. According to Ayurvedic philosophy, they can also be found in various compositions in our body, as they make up each dosha and have an effect on the different functions of the body.

Earth   The solid, material structures of the body (e.g. bones, muscles, teeth).

Water   Bodily fluids (e.g. plasma, sweat, urine).

Fire   Present in the transformative processes of the body (e.g. digestive system, hormones, temperature regulation).

Air   Governing anything that moves (e.g. circulation of blood, breathing, elimination of waste products, flow of thoughts).

Space   Wherever there is space in the systems of the body (e.g. the gastrointestinal tract, the reproductive system, the respiratory system).

Doshas

According to Ayurveda, everything in life contains the five elements (see above) and these combine to form three doshas, which are also present in us and all of life. Doshas can be described as "subtle energies" always moving around and within us. The literal translation of dosha is "that which changes", and it is this change, movement and flux that can lead to imbalances in the body, affected by what is going on in the world, by our lifestyle, by what we eat and drink, by our age, and the seasons.

When we have knowledge of doshas and the elements, we can work to maintain their balance, bringing harmony to mind, body and soul. Read below and see if you can get a sense of how the elements are present in the doshas.

The three doshas are:

Vata   Made up of space and air. This dosha is often dynamic with lots of movement. It's erratic, dry, cold, light, rough, irregular and creative.

Pitta   Made up of fire and water, "pitta" is fast moving and full of vitality. Where there's irritation, sharpness and heat, pitta will be present. Also, look for a slightly oily, greasy texture.

Kapha   Made up of earth and water. Key words we associate with this dosha are "wet", "heavy", "cold" and "unctuous". Slow moving, "kapha" gives things stability and structure.

Chakras

A chakra is a wheel or vortex of energy. We have seven main chakras, positioned on the spinal column, from the base to the crown of the head. Chakras can be blocked or overactive, with both states causing physical and emotional imbalance, which can lead to disease and disharmony. We will explore these as we go through the year, looking at how they affect us and how we can gently bring them back into balance.

Yoga

Yoga is now well known in the West, in many forms. The first evidence of people practising yoga was around 10,000 years ago, and it has been practised ever since, and for good reason – because it works!

With its roots in the Sanskrit word "yug" meaning "to unite", yoga is a system for keeping mind, body and spirit united and balanced, and therefore bringing health and well-being benefits.

It is not necessary to be able to get your leg round the back of your head (though you can if you want to)! You don't need to be naturally bendy or lithe, as any body shape can do yoga. You don't need to be young – you can begin yoga at any age and still benefit. All you need is an open mind and a willingness to give the practices a go.

There are many types of yoga. I like to think there is a style to suit everyone and every body type. Explore, try a few different ones, and find the one that works for you. I practise Dru Yoga, a particularly accessible style that is firmly rooted in traditional yoga; flowing and evolving to suit the needs of our modern world.

The main thing to remember about yoga is that it is not about pain or pushing through any comfort zones. If something hurts or doesn't feel right, on any level, then stop. Listen to your body.

Mudras

The word "mudra" can be loosely translated as a gesture. Sometimes, it's known as a seal or a lock, because we are holding parts of our body - usually the hands - in a particular position. We use mudras in a variety of ways to facilitate healing and wellness. They are thought to influence the flow of energy (see the text on prana, page 15) through the meridians (like blood vessels, but instead of blood they transport prana) of the body. The pressure applied by fingers on different parts of the hands work in a similar way to reflexology or acupressure. In yoga and Ayurvedic traditions, the fingers represent the elements. The little finger represents water; the ring finger, earth; the middle finger, space; the index finger, air; and the thumb, fire. This allows us to make gentle tweaks to our subtle body when we adopt specific mudras, bringing about harmony and balance.

The great thing about mudras is they can be practised anywhere. Whenever you feel you need their help, you can let your hands move into position and work their magic. Just the thing if you are in need of some emotional first aid! In my experience, though, they seem to work better if you do them in a more focused way, sitting quietly and holding for at least five breaths. Some will have an immediate effect, but for longer-lasting results, you may need to practise your chosen mudra regularly over time.

Prana

Put simply, prana is life force. We breathe in prana, but it is more than just the air we breathe. It represents vital energy that flows around and within us.

The Moon

Since ancient times, we have been fascinated by the moon. We track its progress across the night sky, following as it waxes and wanes. We see the effect it has on the ocean's tides and the earth's water tables. As we are approximately 60% water, holistic theory suggests that the moon can also affect us, and has long been associated with our emotions, not always in a positive way. I'm thinking here of the word "lunacy", derived from "lunar", as well as legends associated with the moon, such as werewolves. Many cultures have linked the 29½ day cycle of the moon with the menstrual cycle of women, although there isn't any scientific evidence to confirm this. One thing I have noticed – and hear from others – is that it's more of a challenge to get a good night's sleep around the time of a full moon.

Whether you choose to believe the moon affects you or not is, of course, entirely your decision. I hope you might find it both fun and interesting to explore the ideas presented in the book as we consider the full moons of each month, each one with its own personality.

I hope you have found the above information interesting and that it has inspired you to delve deeper into these fascinating subjects. Let's embark now on our year of wellbeing and discover a treasure trove of wellness ideas.

366 Days
of
Wellbeing

January

1 January

HAPPY NEW YEAR!

Let's start the year as we mean to go on – relaxed and taking the best care of ourselves. No pressure, no strict regimes, just tender loving care for our mind, body and soul. Find some quiet time today to think about how you want the year ahead to look. Here are a few questions you might like to consider:

- What does good health mean to you?
- What would it mean to you if you took the best care of yourself? How would this feel?
- Is there anything you would like to do this year or achieve (maybe it's something you used to do and miss)?

Treat yourself to a beautiful notepad in which you can write, draw or stick pictures of your thoughts, goals and ideas, perhaps even charting your journey through the seasons of the year. It's great to have a reminder of what's important to you and a record of how far you've travelled.

This is your year to shine.

2 January

I like the feeling that comes with a new year – a fresh start and a clean slate. It is like starting a new school exercise book, full of promise and hope.

It's a time of year to reflect and let go of the past, and to think about what we want from life and the year ahead. I believe that bringing some stillness into your day is one of the most beautiful things you can do for yourself. It is an amazing way of tuning into your dreams. The silence that comes with the stillness allows us to quieten the ever-busy, wanting mind, so you can listen to your heart and tune into what you truly want (quite literally, your heart's desire).

How about giving yourself the gift of five minutes (more, if you feel inclined!) of silence and stillness every day? If you feel you can commit to this, you'll find it even more beneficial if you can do it at the same time each day. Try doing it first thing in the morning or last thing at night. It will soon become as much a part of your daily routine as brushing your teeth, and without doubt, you'll notice the difference.

---

3 January

We can often feel depleted at this time of year. The busyness of the festive period – drinking and eating food that might not be the best for us and the long, dark nights – can leave our batteries low. I bet you don't let your phone run out of charge! How about you focus on recharging your personal energy battery before it runs right down? There's no better place to start than by tackling stress.

Stress not only drains our energy levels, it also depletes and weakens our immune system. **Please** take time out, at least once a day, to focus on relaxation. I know this might sound unrealistic or unachievable, but at least consider it. Taking time to relax is never wasted and it's not selfish. It's like being in an aeroplane when the oxygen masks drop down – you must put your mask on first before helping anyone else. Take the time to recharge your battery, so you can give more to others **if** you choose to do so.

Consider how you could create a beautiful, safe space for relaxation. Here are a few ideas:

- Put aside some quiet time. Let it be known that you can't be disturbed (you might need to be creative with this).
- Turn off all media. Maybe put on some soft, relaxing music, or open the window and listen to the birds.
- Make yourself, and the room you are in, warm and comfortable.

- Have everything you need to hand, so you don't have to search for it. You want to make relaxation a simple process.

Let me reiterate...

This is not selfish – this is essential rest.

----

4 January

Why not try this simple relaxation technique today?

- Lie on your back, with your knees bent, if necessary. Lying on your back naturally activates your relaxation response (the parasympathetic nervous system) by pressing on the vagus and sacral nerve plexus, so you are already helping yourself.
- Start to squeeze and release each muscle group. Start at your toes and feet, working up the body. Consciously ask each part of your body to relax as you get to it.
- Curl and stretch out your toes. Push your heels away, then point your toes. Tighten all the muscles through the legs as if drawing the kneecaps up towards your hips, before relaxing. Squeeze your buttock muscles, and release. Lengthen your spine, then press it down towards the earth. Inhale, filling your tummy, then exhale, consciously drawing your tummy in. Now, as you inhale, let the breath extend all the way up from the abdomen into the chest – a full breath – before pausing and letting it go. Draw the shoulder blades together before releasing. Lift your arms slightly from the floor so you can turn them each way, making fists and stretching the palms of your hands out, before letting go. Push the back of your head into the earth to lengthen the neck, then turn the head slowly to each side. Scrunch up your facial muscles before consciously relaxing them.
- Rest in stillness for a few breaths and focus on the gentle rise and fall of your abdomen.
- When you are ready to come out of relaxation, take a couple of deeper breaths. Bring your awareness to your head, shoulders, hips, knees and feet. Then, gently move your body as required – wriggle your toes and fingers, stretch, rock and twist. Roll over onto your right side and, when ready, push up into a sitting position.

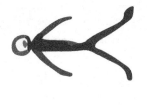

---

5 January

It's great to become familiar with your natural breathing rhythm. The breath is often one of the first things to change when we are stressed or anxious, so this knowledge can be useful for keeping us in balance.

In yoga, we call breathing practices "pranayama". We use pranayama to help bring calm, balance and clarity to mind and body. Whenever pranayama is practised, you need to be relaxed and the breath must never feel forced, rough or strained. So, if you are not comfortable, or if you feel tired or lightheaded, then stop!

The easiest way to get started is to lie on your back with your knees bent. If comfortable to do so, let your knees fall out to each side, so the soles of your feet come together (this allows you to feel the movement of your diaphragm easier). Place your hands on your tummy, with your middle fingers touching just above your navel. Let your breath settle – do not force or try to alter it, just be aware. Once you are in a rhythm, focus on the movement of your abdomen, feeling the tummy rise as you breathe in, with your fingers lifting and separating a little. Your tummy will fall as you breathe out, with your fingers coming back together. You might be able to feel how this breathing rhythm corresponds to the movement of your diaphragm at the bottom of the ribcage. Can you feel the diaphragm flatten and contract as you inhale, with the tummy expanding a little to allow space for the abdominal organs as the diaphragm pushes down? Perhaps it is easier to feel the diaphragm as it moves upwards, pushing the breath out as you exhale, thus allowing the tummy to relax.

You can rest here, focusing on your breathing, for as long as you feel comfortable. Don't be surprised if you find your breath slowing down as you practise.

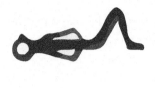

---

6 January

I love to journal. The journal entries are private to me and are done my way. Each day, I detail all kinds of information such as my yoga practice and revelations, "would like to do" lists and things to remember, along with lists of daily gratitude, joy and achievements. In short, everything goes in my daybook! I love to decorate my journals too. I like to get creative, sometimes drawing, designing and writing in different scripts or colours, and sticking in pictures. Every page is different, each one artistic (or so I like to think!) and personal to me. It is a joy to journal and to re-read entries. My journals are a creative outlet in every way.

Is this something you would like to explore? I prefer a beautiful journal, but friends of mine like plain, utilitarian notebooks so they don't feel the pressure to keep them neat. Whatever you choose is the perfect choice for you, and whenever, whatever or however you journal is the perfect way for you. My only piece of advice is that you keep your journal private, which will hopefully reduce self-censorship and allow your true creative nature to flow.

---

7 January

Are you managing to get out in the fresh air? I know it's sometimes a challenge when the days are dark and cold, but it really will make a huge difference to your physical and mental wellbeing if you can get out.

Go for a walk, do some gardening, practise yoga or tai chi, or exercise in your garden or the park. Be creative about when and what you do, just make sure you get out there. Being in nature is good for us on so many levels – here are a few of the biggies:

- Movement and exercise support your immune system by aiding the movement of the lymphatic system.

- It helps us to feel more grounded and connected with the earth which, in turn, helps us to put things into perspective, feel more relaxed and at peace.
- Physical activity releases feel-good endorphins – neurochemicals that not only help us to feel better emotionally but also help us to manage pain.
- If we're lucky and there's a bit of sun, we might be able to top up our vitamin D levels a little – a much-needed nutrient for the immune system.

---

8 January

Have you ever watched a cat or dog after it's had a run-in with another animal or a fright? They give themselves a satisfyingly thorough shake out, and for good reason. It helps them to release any residues of the flight or fight hormones, allowing their muscles to release tension as they bring themselves back into balance. Shaking out breaks the stressful state, signalling to the mind and body that they are now safe and able to relax. We can learn a lot from our wise animal friends.

We do a lot of shaking out in Dru Yoga classes for all the reasons above, as well as to get the body moving a little before we do our postures. We can literally shake off the troubles of the day.

Start by shaking out one hand. This should feel good, dynamic enough that you can feel the release but not so vigorous that you might jar any muscles or joints. Let all your fingers and your wrist relax. Move up into the elbow, then the shoulder, letting the arm feel relaxed and floppy. Shake it all the way through, moving it in different directions if you can. Now let this arm rest and feel the difference, before you repeat the exercise with the other arm. Now to the legs (hold onto something if balance is a challenge). Shake out the foot and ankle of one leg, moving into the lower leg, then the thigh and hip. See if you can shake the leg in different directions – in front, behind and to each side. Place the foot down again and be still for a moment, noticing how it feels. Then swap legs, shaking out from the foot all the way up to the hip. With both feet on the floor, give your whole body a shake. Like a dog that's shaking off water, shake out from snout to tail! I bet you feel more energised now.

9 January

Today, have a think about your comfortable standing position, by practising the "mountain pose". Start by standing with your feet hip-width apart. Have a look at your foot placement. Are your feet and hips happy if you move them so that the big toe is pointing forwards? Soften your knee joints, don't lock them out. Slowly and gently move your pelvis forwards and backwards until you find a comfortable position. It can be helpful to imagine your pelvis as a bowl full of water. If you roll your pelvis one way, the water would pour down the front of your thighs. Roll the other way and it would pour down the back of your thighs. We're aiming for a neutral position, whereby the water stays in the bowl. Now focus on a gentle lengthening of your spine, moving your ribs away from your hips, creating some space at the back of the waist. Allow your sternum to lift slightly. Shrug your shoulders up to your ears, then, consciously, let them relax. Rest your arms by your sides, with your fingers gently curled. Lengthen the back of your neck, with the top of your head uppermost, so your chin is parallel to the floor (you might need to draw your chin in a little).

If you can, stay in this position for a few breaths. How does this feel? Hopefully this gives you a stable yet relaxed base.

With each in-breath, feel yourself rising tall from your firm foundation, feeling the connection you make with the earth on each out-breath.

---

10 January

Here's a leading question...

Do you schedule in your diary downtime, creative time and sleep? Whenever I ask this, the answer is usually accompanied by a rolling of the eyes and snorts of "I wish"!

I know it's hard. Ours is a fast-paced (and getting faster) world, but scheduling time to rejuvenate is essential. Many of us are living with a large sleep debt. Constantly on high alert, we are tired and weary, and the truth is that this will eventually catch up with us. As I've already said, taking time out is never selfish.

A useful little tip I learnt to help prioritise "me time" is to put it in my diary. This is particularly important when I can see I have a busy time ahead, or when I feel the world has had a bit too much of me. I've also learnt that I can't always be trusted, so when I suspect I might ignore my needs, I get a red pen and write next to my diary entry, "Do not cancel – this time is essential for my health and wellbeing".

11 January

Maybe you've seen pictures of people sitting in meditation with their hands in a particular position – elbows resting on their knees, with tips of their first finger connected with tips of their thumbs. This is called "chin" or "jnana" mudra. A mudra is a seal used to harmonise the flow of energy in the body and positively affect our mood. This particular mudra is traditionally used in meditation and is said to create a never-ending circuit of energy and consciousness. When we sit this way, it reminds us that this is our quiet time, a time for reflection, to connect with our higher self. This mudra has many benefits to our emotional body, encouraging us to trust our inner wisdom, calming an agitated mind whilst improving focus, concentration and clarity. It also has some physical benefits, helping us to beat insomnia and strengthen our nervous system. Try holding this mudra for a few minutes in the morning and just before you go to bed. Feel the difference it makes to your mind and body.

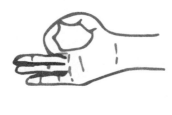

12 January

Here's a great stretch if you have been sitting at your workstation for a long time. Come into standing with feet hip-width apart, feeling that your feet are firmly planted on the earth. You might want to hold onto your chair with your right hand, wherever it reaches, to give you a bit of leverage. As you inhale, lift your left arm up by your ear. Draw the flesh in away from your pants as you exhale. With your next inhalation, feel your spine lengthen and expand as you side-stretch over to the right. Hold for a couple of breaths if you can, feeling your ribs move away from your hips, and your left shoulder easing back so that your chest area opens. Repeat on the other side.

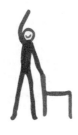

13 January

There are times when I feel like I am being pulled in different directions, leaving me low in energy, feeling scattered and fragmented. As soon as I am aware of feeling this way, I practise this short, effective meditation technique. From sitting, or better still, standing (see 9 January for the beautiful "mountain pose" – the perfect starting point for this meditation), feel the connection you are making with the earth beneath you. Inhale, imagining you are breathing in through the soles of your feet, and let the awareness rise to the middle of your chest – the energetic heart centre. Now let the out-breath travel from the heart up and out through the crown of your head. Draw the next inhalation in through the crown of your head, visualising it travelling down to your heart centre, exhaling from the heart down and out through the feet into the earth. Repeat this process at least three times, keeping your breath relaxed and natural. As I work with this breath, I can feel my spine lengthening and my centre becoming stronger as I call back my energy.

14 January

When it comes to our energy levels and keeping them high, it's a simple equation. The energy we expend has to be less than the energy we take in. If you feel tired, your body is letting you know there's a miscalculation in your energy sums somewhere! The first thing to do is accept that you are tired. Thank your body for letting you know what you need, and maybe take some time to rest. Then consider these two choices:

- Think about how you can expend less energy. For example, taking adequate breaks or doing a relaxation or meditation practice. What can you reschedule or, better still, cancel? Learn to say "no". (Now there's a loaded sentence!) Have some early nights, make time for a siesta, soak in the bath.

Or

- Consider what you can do to refuel. For example, go for a walk, bask in the sun, make sure you are eating nutritious food, have some fun and laugh regularly and heartily, or practise some energising yoga and breathing techniques.

What works for you? Try different things. Make notes in your journal so you can refer to them the next time your battery is feeling flat!

---

15 January

Did you know that each full moon of the year has a name? January's full moon is often referred to as the "wolf moon". There are a couple of theories as to where this name originates, the most common one being that it is a reference to the wolves of North America that howl in the winter months due to hunger.

For me, this moon is symbolic of us shedding the old (i.e. last year) and welcoming the new, and as this moon comes after the winter solstice, it's another sign of light conquering darkness. This is a time for self-reflection, giving thanks and resting, so that we find the energy to be inspired again, able to set new intentions or launch into new projects.

Here are a couple of ideas you might like to try to help you connect with the energy of this beautiful winter wolf moon, whenever it falls this year.

- Go for a walk and enjoy the beauty of a winter's day, regardless of the weather!
- Find some quiet time and maybe embrace some solitary creative pursuits.
- Wolves are pack animals, and the pack is vital for survival. Consider how you can honour or help your pack members (friends, family, neighbours, colleagues), especially the elderly.

- Simplify your day and cut down on the distractions if you can – it's just for one day.

---

16 January

Zzz

According to Ayurvedic wisdom, the body's time for healing is between 10pm and 2am. For optimum healing, start the relaxation process from 9pm so that you are ready to be lying down in bed from 10pm, and you need to be lying down, not sat up reading! I find that early nights are much more tempting when the weather is cold and dark outside, so this is the perfect time for getting into this truly rejuvenating habit.

As the old adage goes, an hour of sleep before midnight is worth two after.

---

17 January

Full of cold? It's certainly the season for it. My suggestion is to try a steam inhalation.

Steam is an inhospitable environment for cold germs, plus the heat and moisture open sinus passages, making breathing easier, as it helps to loosen mucus.

Fill a bowl or the sink with boiling water. Close your eyes and slowly move your head over the steam, about 30cm away. Be careful not to touch the water! Breathe naturally for at least five minutes. You might want to put a towel over your head to trap the steam. Come up for cool air when you need to.

I also like to add a drop of a decongestant essential oil (check contraindications) to the water. My favourites are lavender, peppermint, rosemary and eucalyptus.

18 January

The last thing I want is for my daily sharing to become onerous or preachy. My aim is to help everyone feel the very best they can, which is why I encourage you today to consider the well-known phrase, "you are what you eat". There is so much truth in these words, as the food we eat is turned into the fuel that powers our body. If you are feeling sluggish, lacking energy, or perhaps fighting cold after cold, maybe it's time to look at how you fuel yourself. Think of it this way – just suppose you had a super sports car; would you fill it with basic fuel? I suspect not. I think you would lovingly fill up with premium fuel, knowing this is the way to get the best results, keeping your sports car in tip-top condition for longer. You absolutely deserve the same love and attention...just a different type of fuel!

---

19 January

According to holistic therapies, our kidneys do not like the cold and need a bit more support during winter months. This is perhaps the reason we need to urinate more when we are cold! Here are a few things your kidneys will thank you for this season:

- Keep your lower back and midriff warm by wearing long tops, tucked in.
- Sip on a warming mug of coriander, cumin and fennel tea (see 8 February for more information).
- Stay hydrated. Your urine should be straw-coloured. Darker urine can indicate dehydration.
- Visualise a rich navy-blue colour flowing around the area of your kidneys (either side of the spine, below the ribcage, towards the back of the body). As you practise the colour visualisation, you could also make the sound "shh", saying it quietly or even silently, directing the sound vibration to your kidneys. Feel your kidneys being nourished and rejuvenated as you do this.
- Place the backs of your hands in the middle of your back and warm the area by rubbing gently. Let the hands rest again in the middle of the back, so that you can feel their light pressure. Then, bounce on your heels a dozen times, which has the added bonus of warming you. Shake your legs out to finish, releasing the heaviness.

20 January

Here are a couple of things to be aware of when you move – they will help your body move with ease and grace.

- Feel that all movement originates in the spine, let the movement expand so that arm and leg movements come from their roots, rather than leading with your extremities. This can be particularly helpful to prevent the jarring of muscles and joints, as well as keeping your energy contained.
- When you want to come up, don't just lift. Think about pressing down too. For example, if you lift out of your chair, move your spine and bottom upwards, but also press your feet into the earth to activate your leg muscles, helping to take the pressure off your joints.

Try these movement ideas today – test them, play around with them, and enjoy the feeling of your body moving.

---

21 January

Zzz

Insomnia is a problem for many people (including me at various times in my life) and it has many possible causes. I can't say I have found a magic cure when it comes to insomnia, as I seem to need different things at different times, but what I do have is a large toolbox of tips and techniques. Throughout the year, I'll be sharing some of the things that help me get a restful night's sleep. I always think it's worth going back to basics, so let's start by reminding ourselves of good sleep hygiene practices.

- Get up at the same time every day. Try to also keep a fixed bedtime.
- Allow yourself at least 30 minutes of wind-down time to prepare mind and body for sleep. During this time, dim the lights to stimulate the production of the sleep hormone, melatonin. Unplug all devices that can cause mental stimulation. Use this time to concentrate on activities that are more conducive to sleep, such as gentle yoga or a guided relaxation, a warm bath, reading (nothing too exciting!) or listening to soothing music.
- Cut down on your caffeine and alcohol intake and try not to eat too late.
- Make sure you get some physical exercise during the day. In my experience, people are often tired but too wired to sleep. Physical exercise, done earlier in the day, will help to address this problem.

- You need some exposure to sunlight every day to help you balance your circadian rhythms.
- Obvious, though sometimes neglected, make sure the room you are sleeping in is a good temperature for you. A cool, dark, quiet and comfortable environment is usually the most favourable for sleep.

---

22 January

I have a deceptively challenging exercise for you today! It is well worth the effort though, as it helps to strengthen two of the hip flexor muscles, the "iliacus" and the "psoas", which work as a pair (known as "iliopsoas") as part of our core stability muscles, so can be helpful if you sit a lot during your day.

- Start by sitting on the floor with your legs outstretched (sit on a cushion if this is more comfortable). Let your hands rest on the floor behind to steady you, making sure that your shoulders are relaxed.
- Bend your right knee, so that the right foot is level with your left knee. The right foot isn't touching anything – not the floor, nor the left knee.
- Now open the right hip out, so the right knee is out to the right at an angle of just less than 45 degrees (still not touching the opposite knee or the floor). Hold for 20 seconds if you can, without taking the weight into your shoulders.
- Release and repeat on the left side. Complete three rounds on each side if you feel inclined to do so!
- Your leg and hip may well quiver. This is normal, and you will notice this less as the muscles strengthen.

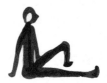

23 January

Yesterday, we focused on strengthening our iliopsoas muscles. These muscles can get very tight, which cannot only cause back pain but have also been linked with heightened anxiety and overall tension. Give this stretch a go. It is particularly helpful if you tend to stick your bottom out!

- Lie on your back on the floor, with knees bent and feet flat to the floor.
- Draw your right knee into your chest, holding round the shin with both hands.
- Push your lower back into the earth, feeling the firm connection you make with the floor. Maintain this connection as you allow your left leg to straighten, sliding it along the floor.
- The moment you feel your lower back leave the earth, stop the left leg sliding. Hold for a breath or two, still gently pressing your right thigh into your chest, as you feel the front of your left thigh/hip soften and relax.
- Release, returning your legs back to the starting position. Then repeat, bringing the left thigh into the chest.

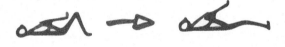

---

24 January

We're always being told to drink more water. What you might not have thought about is the temperature of your water. My tip is to drink your water warm, poured from a freshly boiled kettle and cooled to suit. Warm water aids digestion and soothes the nervous system, and it has even been shown to cut down on the production of mucus, making it especially beneficial during cold and flu season. It can take a little getting used to, but why not try a mug today? Make it your first drink of the day to rehydrate your body after sleep and kick-start your digestive system.

25 January

Have you noticed how thirsty your skin is in winter? My skin loves nothing better than to be nourished with a natural oil, such as grapeseed, almond or jojoba. Even better if I warm it first. You can do this simply by holding the oil in your hands (pour a little into your palm and cup your hands together), bringing it to body temperature before applying it to your body. If you have a bit more time, a more effective way is to place your bottle of oil in a mug or bowl of hot (not boiling) water. It will take 5–10 minutes to warm through – just be mindful of the hot water when you remove the bottle. Enjoy massaging the warm oil into your skin. You'll find it soaks in much easier. Pay extra attention to your joints and really work the oil into them.

---

26 January

I find this an effective and simple way to feel settled and manage anxiety. Stand with your feet hip-width apart, with your big toes pointing forwards. Relax your knees and shoulders, and gently draw the lower abdomen towards the spine, lengthening your spine and the back of your neck. If you feel comfortable to do so, close your eyes. Take time to feel the connection your feet make with the earth. Rock your weight back into your heels without lifting your toes. Now rock forwards, so the weight is in the front of your feet without lifting the heels. Repeat this slowly a couple more times.

Still with your eyes closed, if you can, allow your weight to shift around the outer edges of the feet so you are moving from the ankles in a circular motion, as if on the inside of a giant ice-cream cone. Keep the feet connected to the earth and don't let the toes lift. Circle a couple of times clockwise, then a couple of times anticlockwise. When you've finished, return to a point of stillness and focus once more on the connection your feet make with the earth. Move your awareness to the natural flow of your breath, and the gentle rise and fall of your tummy as you breathe. Return to your day feeling calm and relaxed.

27 January

It can be easy to feel a bit scattered at this time of year. Here are a few things you might find useful to focus on to help you feel more grounded, as they all bring balance to your base or root chakra, "mooladhara". (To find out more about chakras, see the Foundation Principles section in the Introduction.)

- Get outside and walk. I know I've mentioned this already, but it really is good therapy to connect with the natural world and affirm your place on the earth.
- Eat root vegetables in stews and soups. These are good, grounding comfort foods!
- Have some quiet time connecting with the earth. Feel that you are putting roots down into the earth. Feel that you are breathing with the earth.
- Wear red. Red is the colour of the base chakra and can help us to feel safe and secure.
- The gemstone "carnelian" brings balance, courage and trust in oneself.
- If it's OK for you, add a drop of a grounding essential oil such as vetivert, spikenard or patchouli to your bathwater or body cream.
- Try a walking meditation, being mindful of the placement of each foot and feeling the weight roll from heel to toe, one foot at a time, treading lightly on the earth.

---

28 January

Imagine that all **your** thoughts are being broadcast – a little screen above your head where all your thoughts are projected out to the world. Is this an alarming thought? Would it change your thinking? I know it would inspire me to uplift my thoughts! The mind is quite lazy, choosing the easy option – our habitual thought patterns – which is not always that helpful, often formed by past events or future projections, and rarely based in the truth of the present moment. It might take practise (it might take a lot of practise, and this is OK), but we can form new thinking habits. Our thoughts and feelings create our reality, so practise quality thinking and elevate yourself above the melodrama of the mind by choosing the highest.

29 January

Yesterday, I touched on the quality of our thoughts, and how the lazy mind tends to select the most frequent thought regardless of whether it is relevant to the present moment or not (more on this later in the year). When we learn something new, we create neural pathways. The more we use this piece of intelligence or information, the pathway becomes stronger, furrowing a deeper groove, so the information is reinforced. Sometimes this is useful, such as remembering how to drive a car, though sometimes it is not so useful. For example, if we've always been told we are worthless, it becomes more ingrained every time we hear, see or experience something that reinforces this thought. Affirmations can be extremely helpful if we are trying to change thinking, gently coaxing the mind to settle into a new groove. The great thing is, in my experience, you don't have to believe your affirmation. The important thing is that you just say it – a lot. The believing will come. How about this to start us off:

"This year, my thoughts uphold and support me, especially the loving thoughts I have about myself."

---

30 January

I like to start my day with a mug of hot water to rehydrate my body (for all the reasons mentioned earlier in the month), followed by a second mug of hot water into which I put a slice of lemon, a couple of slices of fresh ginger and half a teaspoon of honey. I find this an easy way to stimulate my digestive system and cut through morning mucus...sorry! It's great for my skin, too. In winter, I switch to manuka honey for its antibacterial, antiviral, anti-inflammatory and antioxidant properties. Traditionally, manuka honey is used for soothing sore throats, improving digestive issues and helping wounds to heal. It can be a little pricey, but I think I'm worth it...and I think you are too!

---

31 January

This can be a challenging time of year. Lift your energy and your mood, as well as boosting your circulation, with this simple flow.

- Stand in the "mountain pose" (see 9 January) with hands in a palm-pressed position with the thumbs resting in the centre of the chest.
- Take a full breath in, filling the torso, as you take the arms up and over your head, separating the arms at the top.
- As you breathe out, fold into a forward bend, softening your knees, bringing the hands down, fingers to connect with the earth if they reach.
- Move your hands to the back of the ankles. As you inhale and uncurl into standing (knees bent to support your back), sweep your hands up the back of the legs. Your hands should stop when they reach your lower back. Straighten your legs and open your chest, so you are in a comfortable, gentle back bend.
- Now exhale. Slide your hands back down the back of your legs, as you once more lower into a forward bend, bending the knees.
- The hands move to the front of your body as you inhale, uncurling into standing (knees bent to support your back), with arms up and over as before.
- Repeat this flow a few times. You can increase the speed if it feels good for you.

This flow also awakens your spine. Feel your energy rising as your spine becomes free. You might find your digestive system improves too.

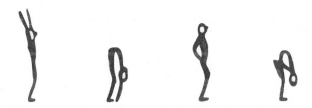

February

1 February

I'll be honest, if I am not mindful of my thoughts and emotions, February can feel quite a tedious month. The prolonged cold, dark and damp take their toll, leading to melancholy, fatigue and weariness. We can add winter bugs into the mix, particularly if we've not taken good care of ourselves. I've learnt to use the days of February to nourish body and soul. We need the energy to help us through the last weeks of winter. Make a list today of things that bring you joy, things that you feel nourish and nurture you and how you would like to feel when spring arrives – these will provide inspiration for you to successfully navigate the end of this chilly season. You might want to pin your list somewhere you can see it. Use it to plan your activities for the month, ensuring you make time for the things that make you feel good.

2 February

Our body is built to move, be it walking, running, jumping, twisting or dancing. Think of all the different ways you can move. We were not designed to sit for hours without shifting position. Here are a few debilitating physical effects our sedentary lifestyles – in particular, sitting for more than eight hours a day – are having on us.

- Decreased leg circulation – your cells are not getting the oxygen and nourishment they need.
- Pressure on the connective tissues and nerves due to compression in the spine and pelvic region. This can lead to back and neck pain, bulging discs, sciatica and repetitive strain injury.

Why not try some of the ways your body moves? How do they feel? What does your body enjoy?

3 February

Building on yesterday's tip about the body's design and desire for movement, how about you set an alarm clock to remind you to get up and stretch regularly? For every hour you sit, move around for five minutes. Get out of your chair, stretch and shake out your limbs. Even better, have a short, brisk walk, or march on the spot! Moving releases built up lactic acid from your muscles (which makes them tense) whilst clearing and refreshing the brain, so you will return to your tasks feeling more focused. We need to move to burn off the stress hormones (adrenaline, noradrenaline and cortisol) which are produced to put us on high alert and help our body and mind deal with potential threat, but continued release of these hormones is debilitating, so do yourself a favour and move. You'll soon feel the difference.

---

4 February

Today, give your circulation a boost with some dynamic twisting. Twisting is great for releasing muscular and emotional tension.

- Stand with your feet shoulder-width apart, bend your knees a little and let your arms hang relaxed by your sides.
- Keep your knees bent as you twist from side to side. Your shoulders should remain relaxed so that your arms hang down like strands of overcooked spaghetti! Then your arms can follow the twisting movement, relaxing the shoulders.
- Bend deeper into the knees each time you twist, so you perform a gentle bounce.
- Move your feet a bit wider apart. If your knees are OK, as you twist to one side, lift the heel of your back foot so you can pivot on the toes, making it a deeper twist. Go steady, so as not to strain or twist your knees.
- Now try lifting the toes of the leading foot, keeping the back heel on the floor as you twist. Allow your arms to swing higher if they will, up and overhead if that feels good.
- Slow the movements down, making them smaller with each twist, until you come to a standstill. Allow yourself to just be. How do you feel now?

5 February

The next time you are in need of calm, or your mind and body require settling, try this simple yet effective gesture. Sit or stand, comfortably. With your palms facing each other, let the tip of the right ring finger connect with the tip of the left ring finger, and the tips of the little fingers to connect, forming a triangle-type shape. Keep this position, holding the hands in front of your abdomen, with the palms facing you. Take a few breaths. Let the hands move up to face the heart centre, still in the same position, again taking a few breaths. Release when you are ready and return to your day with a little more serenity.

The little fingers are said to represent the element of water, and the ring fingers, the earth (read more about this in the Foundation Principles section in the Introduction). So, this mudra helps us to feel grounded and settled, bringing balance to our emotions often connected with the element of water.

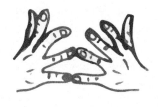

---

6 February

The heavy, damp, cold characteristics of the "kapha" dosha are very much in evidence during winter and as we move into spring. Today, I want to share a couple of simple, practical ideas how we can keep ourselves in balance at this time. We need to get moving to counter the natural still inertia of kapha. Stimulation of mind and body is key. If you feel yourself becoming too sedentary, not wanting to engage, perhaps gaining unwanted weight and sleeping more, these ideas could help you:

- Change your routine, do something different, go somewhere new, meet up with people who stimulate you intellectually.
- Avoid overeating. Choose food that is warm and light, and easy to digest.

- Get active and be dynamic with it! Dancing is the perfect antidote to heavy kapha.
- Learn something new.

---

7 February

The area of the brain that registers smell is closely connected to the area involved with memory. This is the "oldest" part of the brain – the part most developed in our ancestors – and is why perfumes and aromas are powerful triggers of memories and emotions.

In yoga, the sense of smell is associated with the base or first energy centre – the mooladhara chakra (see 27 January for more information). We can harness the energy of this chakra to improve our concentration and memory. Walk out in nature, take time to inhale the fresh air, becoming aware of the earthy smells around you, the scents of the plants, flowers and trees, the smell of the atmosphere. If you do this regularly, you will soon recognise the different smells of each season and how the weather changes the smell of our environment. You may also notice that you gain clarity of mind, and your memory improves.

---

8 February

As we move through the cold and flu season, you might find this infection-fighting drink useful.

Put half a teaspoon each of coriander seeds, cumin seeds and fennel seeds into a flask of boiling water. Allow it to steep for about 15 minutes before removing the seeds. You can keep this nourishing "tea" in the flask to sip at regularly throughout the day.

This is another tool in your kit to support the immune system. I find it also gives a lift when I'm flagging and negates the effects of unsuitable food (worth remembering for party season!).

9 February

It's a good idea to sip at drinks all day long. If you have a foreign body in your throat – microbes such as bacteria or a virus – drinking regularly will help to flush the bug into your digestive system, an important part of our immune system defences, where your stomach acids will kill it. Try the lemon, ginger and honey drink (see 30 January) or the infection-fighting drink from yesterday, to keep your throat lubricated whilst supporting your immune system. Just remember to keep sipping, every 30 minutes or so, throughout the day, and remember warm/body temperature drinks are best.

---

10 February

I don't know about you, but I used to start each new year full of good intentions and resolutions, only to find myself running out of steam round about now... if not sooner!

I hope this little nugget will help take the pressure off. It takes 21 uninterrupted days for a new habit to take root (good habits as well as not so good). As we've already seen, we need to create new neural pathways (see 29 January), so if you are embarking on a new wellbeing habit, or working on changing your thought patterns, go easy on yourself, accept that it will take time and that you will have slip-ups. Everyone does, we are human! Let it go, move on, and continue with your new plan. Don't let your mind drag you into the melodrama of failure or guilt. As the new neural pathways form, it will get easier and easier to stick to your intentions.

Take some time today to focus on all the changes and gains you have already made this year. If you've been working through this book each day from 1 January, why not have a flick through and remind yourself of the tips you have tried? These incremental changes make a huge difference. Let yourself, again, be inspired to take the best care of yourself.

11 February

One of my favourite yoga postures is the "child pose". There doesn't look like there is much to it, but in my experience, it provides comfort and solace when nothing else will do.

Start in a low kneeling position, fold forwards from your hips, so that you are in a soft-rounded seed shape. Let your hands rest along the sides of your body, with your fingers pointing in the same direction as your toes. Alternatively, rest your head on your fists or a cushion if it's more comfortable. You can also modify the pose by placing a cushion between your heels and bottom.

In this folded over position, we can feel safe. Our soft, vulnerable areas are protected, whilst we are showing our harder back/spine to the world. Use it if you are struggling with anxiety. Breathe deeply into your tummy, allowing your shoulders and hips to relax towards the earth. Come out of the fold slowly, uncurling the spine, opening to a new moment.

---

12 February

You've no doubt noticed that rather yukky coating that builds on your tongue overnight. According to Ayurvedic wisdom, this coating contains ama (toxins), a build-up of which can lead to illness, so the daily practice of tongue scraping first thing in the morning is strongly recommended. You can buy proper tongue scrapers for the job, use the tongue scraper on the back of your toothbrush or, failing that, you can **lightly** use the toothbrush itself, gently combing from the back to the front a few times to remove the coating. Remember to rinse your scraper afterwards! It's good to do this first thing in the morning, before you brush your teeth, and before you have anything to eat or drink – you don't want to swallow the ama.

13 February

There is a Sanskrit proverb, "For breath is life and if you breathe well, you will live long on earth". According to ancient yogis – the first people practising and documenting their yoga thousands of years ago – we have a limited number of breaths in our lifetime, and they advise that the way to improve longevity of life is to slow down breathing. Perhaps this has more to do with the fact that slowing the breath down generally leads to less stress, and with it, the associated benefits such as lower blood pressure and improved immunity. I'll leave it for you to decide.

In the meantime, why not sit for a few minutes and let your breath settle, deepening into the abdomen? Once you are in a comfortable rhythm, think about lengthening the out-breath (don't force this), maybe putting in a pause between the inhalation and exhalation (it is a rest, not a holding exercise, so it should feel natural and comfortable, but miss this out if you have heart problems or high blood pressure).

Feel the years drop off you as you relax into this new rhythm!

---

14 February

Today is St. Valentine's Day – a day for love. How much do you consider the love you have for yourself? It has been my sad observation over many years that we are ridiculously hard on ourselves. If we heard someone speaking to a friend or a family member the way we often speak to ourselves, we would be up in arms, and rightly so. Yet, we think it is acceptable to speak to ourselves this way.

Please, on this day of love, take some time for you. Be still and listen to your heart's desire. What do you really need? What steps can you take towards this? Maybe your heart aches for some creative time, a luxurious soak in the bath, sleep, time with loved ones, curling up on the sofa with a good movie, or putting on your dancing shoes. If you don't listen to your heart, you'll never know.

If nothing else, take a moment to read and digest the following quote from the Buddha: "You yourself, as much as anybody in the entire universe, deserve your love and affection."

15 February

February's full moon – the "snow moon" – reminds us that although we are still in winter's icy grip, tiny changes are occurring beneath the earth's surface. We are making tiny changes too.

A full moon always invites reflection. Light a candle, get your journal out and consider the following:

Reflect on how well you are doing – there's no room for criticism, think only of your achievements and qualities. Maybe think about the changes you have made, and the projects or tasks you have started. Positive lists like these are great for reading when you are feeling low.

Show yourself a bit more love too, taking the opportunity to hibernate for a little longer. Make yourself cosy. Enjoy some of your favourite food – choose something that's nourishing and comforting. Settle down with a good read or do something creative. Make the most of these last weeks of winter, and time spent indoors.

---

16 February

My favourite affirmation for February – the month when I most feel I need a lift – is: "I enjoy robust and radiant health."

Short, to the point and it makes me smile. Why not try it today?

---

17 February

How often do you think about your bladder? Chances are not that much until it causes problems! It's never too late to show your pelvic region and bladder some TLC.

Start with some beautiful "butterfly movements". Perfect for men and women, these movements strengthen the pelvic region, improving circulation to the whole pelvic area. Sit on the floor (on a low cushion if you wish), on your sitting bones, with your knees bent and feet on the floor. Start by opening your hips out, keeping the knees bent so that you can bring the soles of the feet together. Lift your ribcage away from your abdomen as your sitting bones connect deeper with the earth, and your hips and knees relax outwards. Focus on the little toe edges of the feet staying together and take time to massage the inner arches of the feet. As you do this, you might just feel your hips relaxing out a little. Keep your ribcage lifted, creating space at the waist and sides of the body. Finish by doing a few rounds of butterflies, by resting your hands on the inner part of your knees. As you inhale, allow the hips to relax, so the knees rise a little. As you exhale, lightly press on your thighs, easing the hips into a more open position, the knees lowering. It should feel comfortable – don't force the knees down.

---

18 February

This lesson took me a long time to learn. I hope you are much quicker on the uptake than I was!

As I mentioned on 3 January, we cannot keep using our energy batteries without topping them up. I hope you've already made a note of things that help you relax. Today, I invite you to take some time out to consider what else you can do to recharge your battery. In my experience, we need different things at different times, so it's worth making a note of everything you find rejuvenating. Here are a few of my favourites – a walk in nature, going to bed early (and even if I can't sleep, resting at least), sometimes eating comfort food, sometimes focusing on lighter food, my yoga practice, having an afternoon lazing on the sofa watching films, time to myself to potter about. I can't think of any better time to plug in and start recharging than a cold and grey February day.

Please take time to recharge regularly. Don't wait until your battery is completely flat.

19 February

Lack of movement, combined with postural weakness caused by sitting a lot, contributes to non-specific back aches and pains. Simple, targeted movements can go a long way to easing the misery of back pain. Here's a great movement to get you started:

Start in an all-fours position, with knees in line with hips and hands in line with shoulders. Your spine should be in a neutral position, so your back is not rounded or dipped. Gently draw the flesh of your lower abdomen, pelvis region and lower back in towards your spine, away from your pants. Hold this steady position without moving your back, breathing naturally all the time. Try to maintain this light abdominal control as you move into and through the "cat posture". On an out-breath, round your back by tucking your tailbone under, pulling your navel in towards your spine and tucking your chin in. As you breathe in, start to put a gentle hollow in the back, extending and lengthening the spine. With your tailbone now pointing towards the back wall, open the chest area and allow the chin to extend forwards slightly. Alternate between these two movements, a beautiful flow easing the back, being careful not to exaggerate the hollowing in the lower back.

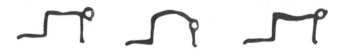

---

20 February

A little earlier in the month (13 February), I invited you to watch your breathing. I hope you got chance to try this and felt yourself relaxing into the rhythm, rather than trying to control it. Watching the breath is a classic way of settling into meditation. Today, let's build on this practice.

Find yourself a comfortable seated position, preferably where you won't be disturbed. Take a couple of deeper breaths, allowing the shoulders to relax. Now let the breath settle, not trying to alter it, just observing the natural rhythm of your breathing. Once you feel this is comfortable (and there really is no hurry) become aware of the feel of the breath as it enters the nostrils. Feel the coolness of the air. Where does it touch the nostrils? Follow its path up to the bridge of the nose. Maybe you can feel the air warming. Now follow the out-breath, from the bridge of the nose, down to the nostrils. Now where do you feel breath on the nostrils? Is it the same place as with the in-breath? Does the out-breath feel different? Allow yourself to become totally immersed in the sensation of the breath, without judgement or any need to change it. Just accept the breath as it is.

Once you become familiar with this technique (again, there's no hurry, this might take minutes, days, weeks or months – there is no competition), you might want to extend your awareness of the breath. Follow its path from the nose into the body and the lungs. Where does the in-breath become the out-breath? Follow its path from the lungs and the body, into the nose and out through the nostrils. Where does the out-breath become the in-breath? Always without judgement, just with the curiosity of an interested observer. Truly, in this moment, nothing else matters.

---

21 February   ⌇ Zzz

Many people find it difficult to relax in our fast-paced world. Sometimes, we need to consciously remind our parasympathetic nervous system (relaxation response) to switch on. I have found these three simple moves very effective at helping many people prepare for relaxation in my work as a yoga tutor.

- Lie on your back. Bring your knees into your chest and hug them, rocking gently from side to side. Draw the knees in towards your chest and hold them there. As you breathe, focus on creating space at the back of your waist. When you are ready, lower the feet to the floor, keeping the knees bent.
- Raise your arms up so your fingers are pointing to the ceiling. Peel your shoulder blades from the earth as you reach your fingers up towards the heavens. Focus on creating space between the shoulder blades. Slowly lower the shoulders back to the earth. Repeat a couple of times if you need to. Try also folding your arms as if you are giving yourself a hug, and again peel the shoulders away from the earth, the elbows rising towards the sky before placing the shoulders back down. Let your arms rest.

- With an out-breath, turn your head to one side, smoothly and gently, with no jerking. Breathing in, the head comes back to the centre. Repeat to the other side, resting when you return your head to the centre. Don't be surprised if you need to yawn at this point!

Now you are ready to go through the squeeze and release relaxation (see 4 January).

---

22 February

Here's a fabulous move, reminding us to engage our core postural muscles, so it will help to support your back as well as help your balance. The firming of the muscles around the abdominal region means your digestive system will love it too!

Grab yourself a cushion or a rolled-up blanket. Sit on the floor, on your bottom, with your knees bent and feet on the floor. Use your hands for support, as necessary. Place your folded cushion or rolled-up blanket lengthways between your legs, so you are holding it in place with your inner thighs. Firm the muscles of the inner thighs, as you are zipping up from the inner knee to the groin. As you do this, notice how you are also engaging the pelvic floor muscles and lower abdominal muscles. Lean back slightly, drawing the lower part of your ribcage in so that it's not jutting out. Remember to keep the inner thighs working! Keep your sternum lifted. Hold for 10-20 seconds. Relax and repeat a couple more times.

Make it a bit more challenging by lifting your feet about 5cm from the floor. Maybe try extending your arms out in front at shoulder-height, instead of having your hands on the floor. You could also lift the lower legs until they are parallel with the floor. Always make sure your inner thighs are feeling it just as much as your abdominal muscles, and check that you are not feeling it straining your back or working your shoulders.

23 February

Have you come across the highly nutritious jam, chyawanprash? Made from amla fruit and 35 different herbs, it has quite an unusual flavour. With its high antioxidant count (one serving is said to provide 35% of our daily antioxidant requirements), it makes a great nutritional addition to your winter diet, as it can help counter seasonal bugs by supporting the immune system. It's also useful if you are convalescing, though is not suitable during pregnancy.

Spread it on your toast as a change to your normal jam. I have a teaspoon of it with my daily porridge. You can even make a nutritious drink by dissolving a teaspoon of chyawanprash in hot water.

---

24 February

I am a huge fan of essential oils. I find them particularly useful when the days are cold, dark and miserable, as they give me a lift. My favourites for this time of year are the citrus scents of sweet orange, bergamot or grapefruit. I put a drop on a tissue and give it a waft when I feel my mood dropping, or I put a couple of drops in a burner to keep me going throughout the day. If I need a boost in the morning, I put a drop on a flannel, placing it in the bottom of the shower tray – the steam releases the heavenly scent. Sometimes, I add a drop of peppermint oil too if I feel I really need waking up, or eucalyptus if my sinuses are blocked. Be sure to check out the health considerations before using essential oils, as they don't suit everyone.

What are your favourite scents at this time of year? Make a note and see how you can use them to bring joy.

---

25 February

Extending from the lower back, through the pelvis, connecting to the thigh bone on each side of the body is the "psoas" muscle. This is one of our hip flexor muscles, used a lot when we are walking or running. We practised some moves last month (22 and 23 January) to help stretch and strengthen this muscle along with its close companion, "iliacus". Let's work a little bit more on this muscle with a simple flow of movements – a great antidote to too much sitting, as well as being a surprising ally when managing stress and tension.

Adopt a runner position. From kneeling, step your left foot forwards, adjusting so that the knee sits over the ankle. Your right knee should stay on the floor, resting on a blanket for comfort. You can also do this from a chair, by sitting on a corner with the right leg stretched behind you. From this position:

- Inhale, sweeping your arms forwards and up, level with your head, opening the front of your body. Exhale, sweeping your arms down and back as you fold forwards over your front knee. With your next inhalation, sweep the arms up and over your head. Hold them here (keep arms low if you have a heart condition), breathing naturally, allowing your spine to lengthen. If comfortable, lift the sternum, firming the tummy a little so that you ease into a slight and gentle back bend, before lowering forwards again on the exhalation.
- From the starting position, extend your arms out to the sides at shoulder-height. Lower your left hand to the floor by the left foot (or rest the hand on the thigh if it feels too much to lower to keep the hand on the floor). Spin your ribs towards the ceiling, so that you can then extend the right arm up into the air. Return to the starting position, then lower the right hand to the inside of the left foot, with the left side of the ribs open upwards towards the ceiling, extending the left arm up into the air (you can always keep the top arm bent at the elbow if it is better for your shoulders).
- Repeat this flow with the right leg forwards.

Once you feel steady with these moves, make them more dynamic by:

- Taking the back knee further back so you feel a wonderful stretch in the front of the hip of the back leg. Keep the knee of the front leg in line with the ankle.
- From the above position, rise onto the toes of the back foot, feeling a gentle push through the heel. Then try lifting the back knee from the floor, just a little way, keeping a low lunge position. Firm up your inner thighs to keep the front knee steady.

Enjoy!

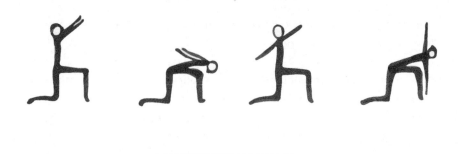

26 February

 Zzz

We can use breathing practices to help trigger our relaxation response. This simple breath ratio exercise works wonders.

You can do this sitting, standing or lying down, it doesn't matter, so long as you are comfortable and feel safe. (It's perfect to do when you're laid in bed, waiting to get to sleep.) Start by establishing a steady breathing rhythm – in for a count of four, out for a count of four. Don't force the breath – it should always feel smooth and nurturing. Once you've anchored this breath and relaxed into it, begin to lengthen the out-breath, slowly and steadily, one count at a time, until you can double the length of the out-breath. Eventually, you'll be breathing in for four and out for eight. Continue with a few more breaths if it feels good. This lengthening of the out-breath will naturally move you into a more relaxed state of being.

Stop if you feel lightheaded or the breath is in any way forced, uncomfortable or feels rough. These breathing practices should always feel easy and sweet.

27 February

♡

There are times when we all feel our world is being rocked, when we lack courage and stability. The next time you feel a need to tap into your inner strength, to build firm foundations from which you can rise tall, try using sound. Slowly and steadily, at whatever volume works for you, vocalise the sound "lam". This sound specifically activates our root/base chakra – the personal energy centre focused on survival and security. At times when you need more calm rather than more strength, use the sound "oo" (as in the word "soothe"). You can repeat these sounds as often as you like, until you feel a shift in your energy.

28 February

Sometimes, our digestion runs too fast...and sometimes it runs too slow. Show your intestines a bit of love with this simple move to encourage the smooth running of your digestive system. It's particularly good for easing a bloated tummy (it releases trapped wind, so you might want to practise in private!).

Lie on your back, keeping your legs outstretched (if comfortable). Should your back need extra support, bend your knees with your feet on the floor. Inhale, bringing your right knee into your chest, taking hold of the shin with both hands. Raise your head from the floor as you exhale. Lower your head on the inhalation. As you exhale, stretch the leg out again along the floor.

Repeat this four times with the right leg and then four times with the left leg, coordinating breath with movement.

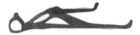 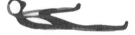

---

29 February

If this is a leap year, then today is a special day – a day of grace. How will you spend it? My greatest wish is that you can spend some time today doing something you love, something that brings joy, something that truly nurtures your mind, body and soul. Maybe you'll have an extra-long soak in the bath with some beautiful nurturing bath goodies. Perhaps you'll practise some yoga or try meditation. How about a walk, connecting with the elements? Find time to explore your creative side. Or how about putting on your favourite movie? Maybe you'll dance to songs that lift your spirit. You could refer to your list from 1 February for inspiration. One thing I would like to assure you of, is that you don't need to do anything at all if you don't feel like it! It's perfectly fine to just rest if you find yourself with some spare time – we don't need to fill every hour. Whatever you find yourself doing with your extra day, enjoy it.

March

1 March

I like the idea of emerging from my winter cocoon like a vibrant caterpillar, shedding my dry and scaly winter skin (physically and metaphorically), ready to soak up all the fresh creative ideas of a new season. Spring is here, meteorologically at least!

Spring is certainly a joyful season, but as it's a tricky transitional season, we need to take a little extra care of ourselves, just as we nurture the first tender shoots of plants. Our winter body is depleted, leaving us less resilient than we otherwise might be. We need to remain vigilant, willing to tweak our self-care tactics, responding to the changing weather – cold and wet one day, gloriously sunny the next. My top tip today is to try to keep your body at an even temperature throughout spring. Keep your layers on so you don't get caught out by the cold, peeling off or adding more as the day dictates. Your body will thank you for it.

2 March

Our mudra (gesture) this month is the "prana" mudra, great for reducing stress levels, whilst also giving a shot of energy. In yoga, prana is life force, so you might've guessed that this mudra is also going to help beat tiredness and fatigue. It is said to give extra support to your immune system too.

Lightly touch the tip of your thumb with the tips of your ring finger and little finger whilst you stretch out the other two fingers. Hold this position, taking a few relaxed breaths. It's recommended you sit or stand whilst doing this mudra, and not to do it whilst lying down.

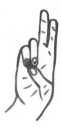

3 March

Spring is traditionally the season for tackling a deep clean of our home. I always enjoy a good clear-out of clutter, opening all the windows and letting the vibrant energy of spring blow the winter cobwebs away. This is a process of lightening up. We can apply the same principles to lighten up our mind and body, with a few simple spring-cleaning lifestyle tweaks. The heavy-holding quality, so important in winter when we need to protect our reserves, is now accumulating dampness and potentially turning stagnant. Just as the snow caps melt, flooding the rivers below, this accumulation of heavy dampness starts to melt within us, leading to spring colds, allergies and tiredness. Now is the time to support our organs of elimination, and our mind. If you are in good health, you might want to consider a short fast – highly recommended in Ayurveda for those with no underlying health conditions. Maybe try cutting down time during the day when you are eating, perhaps eating only between 10am and 6pm. Or fast from the food you know doesn't support you. Peruse the spring-themed tips throughout the next three months, try things out, and see what helps you to feel lighter and revitalised.

4 March

Our bodies have amazing natural barriers, such as the skin and mucous membranes, protecting us from pathogens like bacteria and viruses. Today, let's consider the mucous membranes. Spring is the perfect time to give "jala neti" (saltwater nasal washing) a go. I do this first thing in the morning to clear out any congestion from the night. During hay-fever season, I also flush my nostrils out when I've been out for a walk to get rid of the pollen, whilst in winter I flush them out after I have been with people to wash out any germs I might have picked up!

To practise, you'll need a jala neti pot (a small teapot with a long spout – plastic ones are very reasonable to buy). It might take a little bit of getting used to, but it is well worth it in my opinion. This is not for you if you suffer with nosebleeds, or if you have structural blockages, for example, from a nose break. If your sinuses are very blocked, it might take a few goes to loosen things up. Check with your medical practitioner if you are concerned.

- Add a flat teaspoon of salt (I like rock salt) to 500ml of body temperature water. Stir to dissolve.
- Pour 250ml into your jala neti pot. Lean over a basin, tipping your head on one side, angled slightly down. Place the nozzle into the top nostril and gently start to tip the water through. You'll feel it moving through your sinus passages. Don't be alarmed – it will come out of the other nostril (and if it doesn't – perhaps if there's a blockage – it will just run out of the nostril you've poured into). If it runs straight down the side of your face, you need to angle your head more onto one side and point downwards. The trick is to just go for it, avoiding starting and stopping, which is when you get covered in water.
- When you've emptied the contents of the pot, repeat on the other side with the remaining 250ml.
- Dry the nose by **gently** blowing through both nostrils. Then, close one nostril then the other, gently blowing the open nostril. Now try turning your head on one side, then the other. Finish with your head forwards, closing one nostril then the other.

----

5 March

Let's liven up this early spring day (or indeed any day!) with a dynamic step and swing flow.

Start by anchoring your left foot. Step forwards with your right foot, allowing your arms to swing up, with relaxed shoulders. Lower your arms as you step the right foot back in line with the left. Continue with these movements, settling into a steady rhythm. You might also be able to coordinate these movements with your breath. Inhale as the arms move up, exhale as the arms relax. Come to a stop, then repeat on the other side, anchoring the right foot as you step with your left foot.

If you are feeling dynamic, try switching up with these additions.

- Play around with the arm movements by opening them out to the side, and then perhaps bending the elbows with the palms facing forwards. What feels good for your shoulders?
- Once you are into a relaxed rhythm of swinging the arms, maybe you feel them naturally bend at the elbows as the arms move up and overhead, giving the tops of the shoulders a gentle nudge.
- Instead of stepping the moving leg back into line with the anchored foot, how about stepping it back so you can make a longer stride? You might want to do a double arm movement with this – arms swing up as you step forwards, then lower and rise again as you step back, and so on. Keep your shoulders relaxed so that your arms flow freely.
- If your knees are OK, slow it down as you step forwards and see if you can lower into a lunge position, using your bottom and thigh muscles to lift you back up.

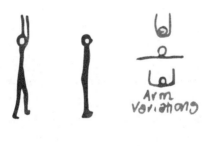

Arm
Variations

---

6 March

Do you know the story of Pandora's box? When all the evils were unleashed into the world, the one thing that was left was hope. You might find yourself today hoping for an end to the cold and damp.

I particularly enjoy my daily dog walks at this time of year, looking for those first tentative signs of spring. I'm always thrilled to see the delicate blossom buds on the trees, pushing away winter's icy grip. Little floral affirmations that spring is on its way, regardless of how cold and wintery it may feel right now. Spring will always follow winter, just as light will follow dark. Remember to look up to the blue of the sky. Remind yourself to focus on the space, not the confusing wood of the trees. Stay positive. Cultivate patience. Our hope for warmer days will be rewarded.

---

7 March

As we leave the heaviness of winter, you might find you are naturally drawn to lighter food in springtime. Go with the wisdom of your body and focus on food that is warming, light and easy to digest. This will help to dry up the excess dampness (mucus) we increasingly find in spring. If the weather turns colder, which it often can in spring, make sure that your diet is keeping you warm. Soups and stews are perfect, including pulses and light grains (e.g. rice, quinoa, millet). Ayurvedic wisdom recommends we favour food that is bitter (e.g. spinach, turmeric, kale, rhubarb), astringent (e.g. broccoli, asparagus, apples, pears) or pungent (e.g. ginger, chilli, radishes) in spring, whilst avoiding too many sweet, sour or salty foods.

---

8 March

Following on from yesterday's tip about spring food choices, here are some other sage words about food (pun intended!). Try to avoid cold and raw food and drink straight from the fridge. These can be too difficult for our digestive system to deal with, potentially extinguishing our already diminished digestive fire that has been weakened during the winter months. I suspect if you listen to your body, you know this. The last thing you really want is a cold salad when the weather is wet and windy – it just doesn't feel nourishing, does it? It's also good to avoid overeating and snacking between meals, both of which can add to the feeling of heaviness at a time when the energy of the season is naturally lighter.

---

9 March

Not everyone finds it easy to relax. When relaxation seems an almost impossible task, try using some props to help you feel safe and secure. Here are a few suggestions:

- Try using a weighted blanket. If you don't have one, throw a couple of blankets or a duvet over yourself for a bit of extra weight.
- Push your feet against the wall.
- Cover your eyes with an eye pillow, or cotton wool pads soaked in rose water.
- Put something soft yet weighted, like beanbags, on the palms of your hands.
- Hold something soothing that represents calm to you. I like smooth pebbles, or maybe a gemstone.
- Use a collection of pillows to prop you up into a semi-reclining position, so that you are more rested than sitting but not lying down, which can feel vulnerable.

Don't be afraid to get creative at relaxation. Do whatever is right for you to get the most from your rest time.

---

10 March

Something I love to do, every day, is put myself in a bubble of bright, healing white light. I focus on every cell of my body being filled with the light, as well as visualising the light encircling my entire body so that I am cocooned in light. I feel the light is nurturing and protecting me, affirming this to myself as I scan through my body. Give it a go. If nothing else, it's a beautiful way to end a relaxation.

---

11 March

Our lymphatic system, a subsidiary circulation system, is a key part of our immunity, transporting leucocyte and lymphocyte cells which "hoover up" bacteria and other debris, as well as taking away any excess waste from the tissues that the blood cannot manage. If the flow of lymph is obstructed, this leads to oedema, where the tissues swell due to the collection of these excess fluids. Ankles are a common area for swelling, as are areas where lymph nodes have been removed, such as under the arm during treatment for breast cancer. **Always get any lumps or swellings checked out by your GP**. Once you know it's nothing serious, you can help yourself and support your immune system by moving around, maybe taking part in regular exercise (put simply, lymph moves when we move) and trying things such as massage and body brushing (see 12 March). In the case of heavy legs from too much standing, I find it beneficial to lie on my back with my legs resting up the wall – you can feel the heaviness quite literally draining away.

12 March

Yesterday, I mentioned how body brushing stimulates lymphatic circulation. If you've not tried it before, spring is an excellent time of year to get into the habit, tying in with our theme of letting go of the heavy, stagnant energies of winter. You can use your hands, but I like to use a soft body brush. Starting at your feet, working your way up your body, lightly sweep your brush or hands upwards, always in the direction of your heart. Brush over your feet, up your legs (front and back), over your hips and bottom. Sweep the mid-section of your body, again in the direction of your heart, before working over the hands and arms, moving towards your armpits. By always sweeping towards the underarms and heart, you are moving the lymphatic fluid back to the heart, from where any toxins that the fluid is carrying can be transferred to the blood, and to the kidneys and liver, for elimination.

13 March

I love the taste of ginger. Its pungent flavour makes it the perfect addition to our spring diet. Ginger has many health-promoting properties for all through the year. Said to be anti-inflammatory, it has long been used as an aid for digestion, easing cramps and digestive upsets, in particular nausea. We've also seen that it cuts through mucus, so it's useful during both cold and hay-fever seasons. As well as eating and drinking ginger, it can also be applied as a soothing poultice. Soak a cloth in warm ginger tea and wring it out before applying it to your lower abdomen. If you like a bit more warmth, use a hot water bottle too, which can be just the thing for alleviating menstrual cramps or a griping tummy.

14 March

One of my favourite yoga postures for cold, damp days is called "the fish". I have found it to be an amazing posture for supporting my immune system. As it stretches the chest and groin areas, it helps with the drainage of lymph, plus it is said to stimulate the thymus gland, which produces important immune cells. It's also soothing and relaxing, so another tick in the immune support box! Here is a modified version of the full yoga pose, which is easy for everyone to practise. Oh, and it's also good for easing a stiff back.

- Lie on your back, with knees bent and arms to your side with palms down.
- Exhale, pressing your back into the earth.
- Inhale as you arch your spine away from the earth, keeping your bottom on the floor.
- Flow between these two moves. As you relax into the posture, draw your shoulder blades a little closer together as you inhale, so you feel a gentle lift in your chest area.
- To finish, bring your knees into your chest and rock gently.

---

15 March

March brings the last full moon of winter. As the earth warms and softens, awakening from its deep sleep, earthworms start to rise to the surface, giving our "worm moon" its name. It is a time for new beginnings, hope and optimism as we shake off the old, stagnant, holding energy of winter.

Although you might be enthusiastic about your spring projects, don't overdo it and burnout before you've returned to full vibrancy. Think about what you can simplify in your life and home in on a few important things, being realistic about what you can do, so that you do not spread yourself too thin.

You might want to plant some seedlings too - a visual reminder of the creative potential of the season.

16 March

Medical studies have linked good balance with improved brain function and health, finding that people who are able to stand on one leg for 20 seconds were less likely to develop conditions such as dementia. It's also known that improving balance reduces the incidence of falls, as well as having a beneficial knock-on effect on the overall strength and health of our back and joints, as we work these muscles when we are balancing.

Try this simple exercise a couple of times a day, for the next week, and I bet you notice an improvement.

- Stand close to a table or kitchen worktop, so that you can hold on if you need to.
- Take your weight onto your right foot, bend the left knee, and see if you can rest just the toes of the left foot on the floor.
- Hold this for about 20 seconds, feeling yourself rise tall from your firm foundations, your leg, hip and buttock muscles gently engaging, feeling your ribcage lifting away from your hips.
- Release and repeat on the other side.
- As your balance improves, try bringing the foot a little higher, perhaps resting it on the ankle, or a bit higher on the calf. Maybe you can release your grip from the table, though have your fingers hovering over the worktop, just in case.

---

17 March

Zzz

Have you ever noticed how busy your mind is in the middle of the night? The trick to taming a monkey mind is to give it something to do. Left to its own devices, the mind will usually end up making mischief, fascinating itself with an endless round of melodramas, thoughts, criticisms and anxieties. When I find myself awake with a busy mind, I always turn to this practice to break the thought cycle. I choose an easy category, such as countries, animals or names – you get the idea. Then, starting at "A", I think of an example for each letter of the alphabet – antelope, badger, cat, dog, elephant and so on. I rarely get past kangaroo before the cycle of thoughts has been broken and I've drifted back off to sleep.

18 March

Flowing with and adapting to change is a useful skill to learn. At times when you feel stuck, help yourself to loosen up and flow with these simple ways to connect with your sacral chakra, "svadisthana". Working on this chakra also has the added benefit of bringing balance to our emotions, whilst encouraging us to tap into our creative side.

- Practise being still – this might take some practise, and this is OK. You'll never be able to force yourself into stillness and this is part of this practice, so surrender and go with the flow.
- Use journalling to get in touch with your inner self. Allow yourself to dream. What do you truly desire?
- Have some quiet time connecting with water. Imagine a calm body of water if you cannot see one. Allow yourself to be absorbed by the ebb and flow, watching the ripples across the surface.
- Wear orange, the colour of the sacral chakra, helping us to go with the flow and be flexible.
- Moonstone and aquamarine gemstones bring balance, whilst emerald gemstones bring calm – useful if you are feeling overwrought and emotional.
- If it's OK for you to use, add a drop of one of these essential oils to your bathwater or body cream – fragrant and feminine, ylang-ylang or rose; cypress to help you flow with life; clary sage for its ability to help you reach a meditative or dream-like state.
- Focus on movements that are fluid and flowing, particularly working the hips and pelvic girdle. Yoga, tai chi and dance are perfect. Water babies might like swimming or taking part in water sports.

---

19 March

How are you at getting out of bed in a morning? Me? Not so good! In spring, though, I feel the difference when I am able to prise myself out of bed before 7am. I find that I have more energy and generally feel lighter. Sleeping in after 7am can leave us feeling sluggish and thick-headed, as well as increase mucus levels, as it aggravates the damp, heavy kapha dosha. Apparently, it's even better if you can rise with the sun, something I've not quite managed every day just yet – I remain a work in progress!

20 March

Got a pain in the neck from sitting in front of a screen too long? Try this easy move for releasing tense neck muscles.

Interlace your fingers and place them on top of your head, with palms down. Press the hands down onto the top of your head at the same time as you push the head up into the hands. You should be able to feel your spine lengthening and your shoulders dropping as you do this. Hold for a few seconds.

Now repeat the move with your hands at the back of your head, gently pushing your hands into your head and the head back into your hands. As you lengthen the cervical vertebrae of the neck, feel the chin subtly moving towards the spine. Hold again for a few seconds before releasing.

---

21 March

As a meditation teacher of many years, I get plenty of questions about meditation. People often consider meditation to be difficult, with complicated rituals, or they believe it to be a mysterious practice and out of their reach. Let me bust the most common myths I hear.

Myth: You have to sit cross-legged in the lotus position, on the floor, for hours.
Truth: You don't need to sit for hours. In fact, sometimes you don't need to sit at all. You can sit on a chair or a stool, or you can do a moving or standing meditation. Continuity is more important, and far more beneficial. Better to sit for five or 10 minutes at a time, regularly (daily if you can), rather than trying to do an hour-long meditation once in a blue moon, or even worse, doing it once and finding it uncomfortable and so never doing it again!

Myth: I'm rubbish at meditation, my mind never stops.
Truth: You will never stop the mind from thinking, that is its job. Our aim in meditation is to increase the space between the thoughts, and when the thoughts do come, which they will, to not get distracted by them, to just let them pass. The more you practise meditation, the easier this will become.

Myth: I can't meditate, I can't sit still.

Truth: Hmm, I wonder how you could get better at sitting. Could it be with practise?! We all have to start somewhere – how about today? Settle yourself down and enjoy a few moments of stillness, watching your breath (see 13 and 20 February).

---

22 March

If you struggle switching your mind off at bedtime, try turning your electrical devices off and stop checking your phone at least an hour before you go to bed. This is not only a signal to the brain that the working day is over, but it also helps to reduce our stress levels so that we are ready for sleep. The blue light that our phones and screens emit, along with the flickering of the screen, put our minds in a state of stress, heightening all our responses, thus making it harder for us to relax in preparation for sleep. If you want to switch off, then make sure you switch off!

---

23 March

Pay your large intestines some extra TLC today, with a variation of the "child pose" (see 11 February). Come into a kneeling position. Resting the hands into your lap, make a soft fist with one hand, wrapping your other hand around it. Now fold forwards into that beautiful child posture, resting your head on a cushion if you need to. Feel the fists create a slight pressure in the abdomen as you breathe (don't push the fists into your body – your body relaxes around the fists). It might not feel too comfortable if you are suffering from constipation or trapped wind, but it is this pressure that is aiding your digestive system, causing a little bit of intra-abdominal pressure. Breathe. See if you can relax into it.

24 March

When we start a new practice, it's all exciting and shiny. You could say we are in the honeymoon phase, so enjoy it! Don't be surprised if one day you fall out of love with your new practice though! This is normal, nothing more than a play of the mind. Watch out for boredom, apathy, frustration and other disgruntles. Again, all are just plays of the mind to throw you off course. The mind and the ego love melodrama, they are not too keen on the peace and calm we are focusing on in our daily tips, usually kicking up a fuss when we are making progress. My advice is to keep on doing what you're doing, ignore what your mind is telling you and listen to the wisdom of your heart.

---

25 March

Earlier in the month, I gave you some ideas of how to release tension from your neck. You might want to add in these movements to help keep your neck muscles healthy.

Sitting or standing, gently draw the flesh away from your pants, and lengthen your spine to support your neck. Keep this engagement throughout the three exercises.

- Start by looking forwards, then lower your chin (don't push it towards the chest, we don't want to strain). Now draw the chin in slightly as you stack the neck vertebrae one on top of the other, uncurling so that you are looking forwards again, feeling a subtle and pleasing stretch in the back of the neck. Repeat this movement twice more – it's almost like you are describing a small circle with your chin.
- From the starting position of looking forwards, this time turn your head slowly and smoothly to one side, with no jerking. Try not to involve your shoulders in the move, it's just the neck. Bring it back to the centre, then turn to look to the other side, and back. Do this twice more. Turn your head on the out-breath, back to the centre with the in-breath.
- Now with your out-breath, from the starting position looking forwards, tilt your head to the side, so that your right ear moves towards the right shoulder. Try not to move your shoulders. Breathe in as you lift back to the centre, before easing the left ear to the left shoulder, and back up. Repeat twice more on each side.

26 March

There are many benefits to getting out for a brisk walk, physical and emotional, including supporting the immune system by boosting circulation, and helping us feel uplifted and more positive. It also shifts the stagnation and heaviness of winter, along with the dampness that tends to increase in our bodies during the spring. Really stride out when you walk, swing your arms, get your heart rate up, so that you are a little breathless, but can still hold a conversation. As we know, spring can be very changeable, so be prepared. Even when the sun is out in spring, it can still turn cold. Your physical body, in particular the head, will not appreciate getting cold, so make sure you have something warm and waterproof to put on in case the weather turns when you are out. Apologies for sounding like your nan but, honestly, your body will be grateful!

---

27 March

Following on from yesterday's tip, I hope you've found time to go out for a brisk walk. There's something rejuvenating about being out in the elements, and focusing on our senses is a great way of connecting with them. The next time you are outside, maybe walking or perhaps sitting by an open window, focus on each of your senses, one at a time. The feel of the atmosphere against your skin, the sounds you can hear, the scents around you, maybe you can taste the atmosphere on your lips. What can you see with soft, relaxed eyes? Give your mind the permission and opportunity to rest.

Affirm your connection with the elements and the senses, enjoying the sensations of each one. For example:

"I am enjoying the feeling of the fresh breeze against my skin."
"I am enjoying the sounds of nature all around me."

Be truly present in the moment, moving beyond judgement to acceptance.

This is a beautiful practice to do with each of the seasons, noting how your experience and appreciation change as you flow through the year.

28 March

Do you remember back in February (see 19 February) I shared the beautiful back-loving "cat posture"? I hope you've had chance to practise it and are feeling some of its benefits. Today, let's build on it and introduce a wave-like flow through the spine. Not only does this help to improve the segmental flexibility of your spine (great if your back is stiff), but in my experience it also improves the flexibility of the mind. We become less rigid in our thinking, better able to navigate a smooth path through the vagaries of life.

As before, start in an all-fours position, with knees in line with hips and hands in line with shoulders. As you flow between the two movements of gently rounding the back as you exhale and lengthening the spine, opening the chest as you inhale, focus on each movement always starting at the base of the spine. Allow the movement to flow like a wave all the way up your spine, your head being the last thing to move. How many of your vertebrae do you feel moving independently? Are there some segments of stiffness? Try the movement, visualising a stream of light flowing up the spine. Let it work into the areas of stiffness, easing out the tension.

---

29 March

Words have such power – the power to truly uplift or the power to deeply wound. Often, words are spoken without much consideration as to how they might be received or the impact they might have, and sadly, once uttered, our words cannot be taken back. Perhaps we wouldn't have so many regrets and upsets if we heeded the advice of this beautiful quote before speaking: "Is it kind, is it true, does it improve on silence?"

I like to turn this into an affirmation, reminding me to engage my brain before I engage my mouth. "My words are kind and truthful, uplifting to all who hear them."

Remember, this wisdom applies just as equally to the words you speak to yourself.

30 March

Today, I have a beautiful breathing exercise that encourages us to use our diaphragm correctly and use the full capacity of our lungs. "Pigeon breath" can be done from sitting or standing.

- Let your hands rest under your chin with interlaced fingers, with your arms relaxed.
- Inhale through your nose, lifting your elbows high.
- Exhale through your mouth, bringing your arms together, as you gently extend the back of your neck, with a soft lift of your chin – this is different to tipping the head back (stay looking forwards if you have epilepsy or a whiplash injury). As you breathe out through your mouth, make a soft "O" shape with your mouth, so the breath leaves with a gentle cooing sound.
- Hold this position as you breathe in through your nose. The forearms should be close together and the wrists relaxed.
- Relax your arms (keeping them in position with the hands under the chin). Your head returns to look forwards as you breathe out through your nose. This is one round.
- Build up to five rounds if you can. When you have completed your rounds, relax your arms to your sides and be still. What do you notice about your breath now? Has it slowed down, does it feel deeper, does it almost feel like you don't need to breathe?

IN   IN   OUT   IN

31 March

Do you remember the simple abdominal focus we did at the beginning of the year (see 5 January), to help us get into our natural breathing rhythm and use our diaphragm properly? We're going to expand on this today, and it follows on perfectly from yesterday's "pigeon breath".

As before, the easiest way to get started is to lie on your back with your knees bent. If comfortable, let your knees fall out to each side so that the soles of your feet come together (this allows you to feel the movement of your diaphragm easier, but do bring your knees up if this isn't comfortable). This breathing exercise can be done sitting or standing.

Place your hands on your tummy, with your middle fingers touching just above your navel. Let your breath settle, not forcing it or trying to alter the breath, just being aware. Breathe in and out through your nose. Once you are in a rhythm, focus on the movement of your abdomen, feeling the tummy rise as you breathe in, your fingers lifting and separating a little. The tummy falls as you breathe out, with the fingers coming back together.

Once you feel relaxed with this, bring your hands to rest on your ribcage (the hands no longer need to touch). Inhale and feel the gentle rise of the tummy. Let the breath rise into the rib area, feeling it gently expanding, the hands gently lifting with the expansion of the ribcage. As you exhale, let the tummy relax, then the ribs gently fall. Once you are in a comfortable rhythm, feel the breath rising from the tummy, into the ribs, and finally into the chest. Don't worry if you can't feel the breath coming all the way to the top, just have an awareness of the breath filling your torso - tummy, ribs, chest - it will come as the lungs become used to the movement. Exhale, relaxing the tummy, ribs and chest. Continue with this full yogic breath for as long as you feel comfortable. Remember, it should always feel smooth and relaxed, never forced or rough.

Take your time. There really is no hurry in practising this breath. It is worth the effort, helping to bring calm and clarity, and strength to your lungs.

April

1 April

Spring is a time of rising energy, a time for creativity and joy. Today, take a moment (at least a moment!) to look at the luscious buds on the trees, the beautiful greens of young shoots and leaves, the glorious display of colourful spring flowers. Listen to the birds joyfully singing, their love for the season very clear to hear. Let your fingers gently caress the bark of a tree, the coolness of the grass or soft downy leaves. Maybe you can feel the elements against your skin. How does spring smell – the grass, flowers, trees? Can you taste the newness? This is Mother Nature in all her creative glory, full of promise. Let this energy fill every cell of your body, be revitalised by all that you see, hear, smell, taste and touch.

2 April

It's not always easy to get outside. Perhaps like me you live in an urban area, dreaming of the sea or greener pastures. If this resonates, then bring nature to you! Make your relaxation, living or working areas prana-filled havens of natural beauty. I always like to be able to see some flowers or a plant when I'm working. I also have something beautiful and tactile to hand, like a gemstone or a smooth pebble from my favourite beach, soothing to hold when I'm on the phone or thinking. Maybe your thing is driftwood, pinecones, seashells, conkers, leaves – you can get really creative with this, changing your display with the seasons. Perhaps a piece of artwork will transport you to the great outdoors whenever you look at it. Try a natural sound playlist or hang a wind chime. Is it possible to have a bird feeder close to your window so that you can drift for a few moments, watching the birds go about their business? Make the most of Mother Nature's gifts for an instant mood and energy boost – a chance to reconnect with the world and the elements.

3 April

Today, I have the perfect mudra for spring as it supports new beginnings - the "apana" mudra. It also helps us have an internal spring clean of mind and body, stimulating the clearing out of waste products and unhelpful thought patterns. The energy of this mudra is all about letting go. Give this a miss if you have colitis or IBS symptoms.

I have found this a useful mudra for restoring harmony when I've felt out of sync with the world. You know the feeling, when you are travelling in one direction, whilst the rest of the world is going in a different direction and nobody seems to understand the map you are following!

On each hand, bring the top of the thumb to connect with the middle and ring fingers. Extend the little and index fingers. You can rest your hands in your lap, or let them rest by your side, building up to five minutes, breathing naturally as you hold the mudra.

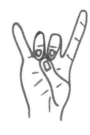

---

4 April Zzz ♡

Hopefully, you have got into rising earlier as the mornings become lighter. It's a good idea to be in bed a little earlier in the spring too, to make sure you are still getting all the sleep you need. Remember, spring can be tricky to negotiate - we need to protect our delicate body as it emerges from its winter hibernation. Aim for "lights out" before 11pm. Apart from a rejuvenating relaxation (keep it short and sweet), it's best to avoid napping during the day, if you can. In spring, I still have my afternoon siesta, but I make myself a little less cosy, so that I'm focused on the relaxation and not so tempted to nod off!

5 April

Enliven your body today with some gentle tapping, a massage technique known as "Do-In". With light fists, tap your muscles, working systematically around the body. Start by tapping on the left hand, up the left arm and round the shoulder a couple of times, swapping to the right arm. Work into the underarm area, too. Tap across your chest and collarbones. Use your fingers to massage down the breastbone (great for clearing congestion in your chest). Tap lightly around the ribcage, seeing if you can reach the sides and round the back as well. Now onto the abdomen, moving up the right side of the tummy, across by your navel and down the left side, always moving in this clockwise direction so you are working with your digestive system. Move onto your bottom, around your hips, down the outside of your legs, onto the feet and up the inside of the legs, repeating a couple of times, before moving down the front of the legs and up the back of the legs. Then, using your fingertips, tap around your skull and down the back of your neck. To relax, give yourself a bit of a shake out when you've finished.

I love how this technique uplifts and warms me. I know it improves the blood circulation to my muscles and joints, whilst also supporting my lymphatic system.

---

6 April

One of the first things to suffer when we are stressed is our digestive system. When we are in a fight, flight or freeze response, our body considers our digestion to be unimportant as it will not help us in this immediate stressful moment. Unfortunately, we are not so great at switching off this stress response and so we suffer with indigestion, upset stomachs, IBS and a whole host of digestive issues, all exacerbated by stress. Here are a few ideas to help you digest life and food a little easier.

- Take time to sit down to eat your meal.
- Be present at your mealtimes. Turn off the TV, put away your phone. Focus on the food and the act of eating – enjoy the food.
- Take a few deep breaths before you eat, lengthening the out-breath, to help you relax.
- Chew your food properly. This is where digestion starts. Remember, your stomach doesn't have teeth!

- Avoid overeating, which overloads your digestive system. Eat mindfully. Eat to nourish.
- If you need a drink whilst eating, try sipping a little warm water. This should be enough to soften the food without putting out the digestive fire.

---

7 April

Today, I ask you to consider how you prepare and eat your food. Food prepared and eaten in a hurry always gives me indigestion and somehow doesn't feel as nourishing, as if it has picked up all the fraught energy. Yesterday, I touched on how stress impacts our digestive system, with stress and anxiety impairing our ability to assimilate and eliminate the food we eat. Conversely, when we eat in a calm and relaxed manner, we feel more nourished and satisfied on every level. Slow down and savour. Eat with awareness. Consciously chew your food. This is the best way to start the digestive process, starting with the taste buds, which activate the salivary glands, stimulating the first stage of digestion. Plus, it gives your digestive organs sufficient time to let your mind know when you are full.

As always, I like to harness the power of my thoughts to help my body. Giving gratitude for the food you have, all the people involved in its production and preparation, and thanking your amazing digestive system, is a beautiful thing to do. This encourages me to take my time, to think a bit more about the food I am eating, so I am eating with awareness, in a relaxed manner, rather than gulping down my meal. Maybe try an affirmation too, perhaps something like "I enjoy the food, which nourishes and supports me on every level. My digestive system works smoothly and efficiently."

Bon appétit!

---

8 April

A favourite springtime yoga posture of mine is the "fig tree". A beautiful balancing pose, which mysteriously helps to clear the sinuses and supports the lungs. As it's a posture that tests your balance, it's also grounding, making it perfect for bringing you into the present moment.

- Start in the "mountain pose". At this point, I like to check in with my breathing, noticing how easy it is to breathe.
- Step your right foot back a little, so you can rest on the toes (keep the foot flat if you are struggling with balance). Let your right arm come out to the side at shoulder-height with your palm facing down. Your left arm stretches up by your left ear, with your palm facing forward (keep the arm down by your side if you have heart problems or high blood pressure).
- Hold this position, connecting with the earth through your supporting leg and foot on the out-breath. Lengthen and expand through your spine with the in-breath (shoulders remain relaxed).
- If you feel steady, see if you can lift your back foot just a couple of centimetres from the floor, keeping the leg straight, without leaning forwards.
- Take your time with the balance, keeping your toes on the floor until you feel steady enough to lift the back foot. It's fine to keep the toes on the floor, you'll get more from the posture by being balanced and steady.
- Bring yourself back into the "mountain pose", before repeating with the left leg back and left arm out to the side.

Notice how quickly you come to a still point – always a good way of checking in with yourself. Once you've completed the posture on both sides, take a moment to become still again with both feet on the floor, bringing your awareness to your breath. Is it clearer, easier or smoother than when you checked in with your breath at the beginning of the posture?

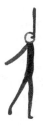

9 April

There's little point slathering on moisturising creams and oils if the skin you are rubbing into is dead! There are many different body scrubs on the market, but maybe you'd like to make your own?

Mix two-thirds of sea salt and one-third of oil (olive or almond oil work well). Add to this a couple of drops of your favourite essential oil, and maybe the zest of something citrusy. Gently scrub all over your body, paying extra attention to dry spots such as elbows, knees and heels, before rinsing off. Now massage in your beautiful moisturiser. Don't be surprised if your skin drinks it in – you'll quite literally feel the difference.

---

10 April

We all know that working on a keyboard all day can put a lot of strain on our back, neck and shoulders, but if you also finish your working day with aching wrists and hands, give this short sequence of moves a try. Do them whenever you feel you need a break, and especially when you've packed away your keyboard for the day.

- Give your hands a good shake out until they feel limp.
- Make fists, then slowly release, stretching all your fingers out wide.
- Circle your wrists in both directions.
- Interlace your fingers. Circle the right wrist a few times in both directions, then do the same with the left wrist.
- Wrap one hand around the opposite wrist. Squeeze lightly, then release. The gentle pressure should feel good. Repeat with the other hand and wrist.
- Finish by shaking your hands out again, allowing that relaxing move to work all the way up through the arms to the shoulders.

---

11 April

Staying in the same position is one of the biggest causes of back pain. NICE (National Institute for Health and Care Excellence) recommends stretching, strengthening and yoga exercises as the first steps in managing lower back pain, and with good reason – there is plenty of evidence on the benefits of yoga in relation to back care. In yoga, we use mindful stretching and strengthening exercises, targeting the core and postural muscles, whilst the relaxation and breathing elements of the practice help us to relax tense muscles and manage pain.

Here is a core strengthening exercise you can try at home. It is best done a couple of times a day, if possible. Slowly build up, and never tolerate strain or discomfort.

- Lie on the floor, on your back, with knees bent and your feet flat to the floor. Your arms should be by your sides, with palms down so you can use them for support, if needed.
- Place a cushion between your thighs, running from groin to knee. Squeeze the cushion firmly with your inner thigh muscles.
- Draw your navel in towards your spine and your pelvic floor up towards the base of the spine. Keep the natural, relaxed arch in the lower back, with inner thighs still working.
- If possible, without flattening the lower back to the floor and keeping all the muscles working as above, lift the feet a couple of centimetres off the floor.
- Hold this, breathing naturally for five breaths, if you can.
- Release and repeat twice more.

---

12 April

You might have seen some natural remedies for hay fever, which involve rubbing a little balm in the nostrils to act as a barrier, helping to prevent pollen and other impurities making their way into the respiratory system. In Ayurveda, there is a similar practice called "nasya", where oil is used to protect and hydrate the nostrils and the sinuses. Not only is it great to do during hay-fever season, but it also helps to keep your nostrils in tip-top condition during the cold winter months, when the harsh weather can dry out the sensitive skin of the nose. I also find it curiously calming, especially around times of change.

The traditional way to do this is to lie on your back and drip in special nasya oil, but an easier, more accessible way is to place drops of nasya oil (coconut oil is a good alternative) onto a clean finger, then gently massage it into the insides of your nostrils.

13 April

Today, I write in praise of a morning routine, a good way to set you up for the day ahead.

- Take a few deep breaths to let yourself come round, giving thanks that you are here to greet another day!
- Have a big yawn and a stretch – it starts to shift the heaviness that might have accumulated through the night.
- Remember to clean your tongue when you brush your teeth (see 12 February).
- Make your first drink a mug of hot water, to kick-start your digestive system and rehydrate, replenishing the fluids lost during the night.
- Before your shower, oil your body, allowing it to soak in before you wash. Mustard oil is warming, coconut oil is cooling, and the Ayurvedic "mahanaryan oil" is perfect for hydrating dry skin and creaking joints.
- If you do it, wash out your nostrils with the saltwater wash (see 4 March) and apply a little oil to the insides of your nostrils, as described yesterday.
- Now you're ready to get moving – maybe a walk or some yoga or tai chi, releasing any residual tiredness, or perhaps sitting quietly for a peaceful start, if you've time, before your breakfast!

---

14 April

Our lungs need a little more tender loving care during spring, according to Ayurvedic teachings. Here are a few ideas to support these vital organs, all tips I regularly use myself, as my lungs love a bit more attention than most.

- Take a moment to be still. Visualise your lungs (find a picture of the position and shape of the lungs if this helps you to visualise them better). Now imagine each time you inhale you are drawing into the lungs the most beautiful, vibrant white light. This light is healing and soothing. Let it fill every cell.
- Avoid mucus-forming food, such as dairy, sugar and wheat.
- Make a gentle "shh" sound, as if asking someone to be quiet. I find this helps me to breathe more easily, less in my upper chest.

- We are said to hold grief and sadness in our lungs. If you have a lung problem, frequent chest infections and the like, consider if this could be the case for you. You might want to journal about this. Seek help if you feel unable to deal with this alone.
- Use affirmations such as "I breathe easily", "I breathe in joy, I breathe out sadness" and "I enjoy the fullness of life".
- Remember to use the breathing techniques I share in this book – they really do work!

---

15 April

Spring is here, and our full moon is named after the delicate pink blooms of wildflowers, the "pink moon".

Autumn encourages us to let go of the past. In winter, we think about our heart's desires, contemplating our goals and intentions, moving them forwards as we flow through spring. The energy of the pink moon gives us the courage and creative impetus we need to pursue our dreams. Tap into this wisdom with a moonlight stroll or a quiet meditation.

Now is also the time to consider our boundaries. As we head towards summer, there are going to be a lot of things that call to us! Events, activities, projects and social engagements, all vying for our attention. It's easy to spread ourselves too thin and burnout. Think about what is important, what you really want to do, and where you might need to set boundaries. These are all great questions for your journal.

---

16 April

Do you ever feel you've lost your zest for life or are feeling stifled, creatively? You might benefit from some sacral chakra exploration. Located in the lower abdomen below the navel, in the area of the perineum, this is our energy centre where we can tap into our creativity, as well as our capacity for pleasure. An easy way for us to connect with this centre, perhaps at a time when we need to find some joy in life or are feeling blocked creatively, is to voice the sound "vam", slowly and steadily.

At other times, when we find ourselves overwrought, we need to calm this centre. Try a few rounds vocalising the sound "oh", again, slowly and steadily, through lips gently rounded into an "O" shape.

---

17 April

Today, I share a simple technique a reflexologist friend shared with me, to help me stay calm. I also find it keeps my hands still, which tend to fidget when I'm anxious. The simple act of keeping my hands still helps me to feel more in control. Cup the left hand in the right hand, with both palms facing upwards. Then, place the thumb of the right hand in the centre of the left palm and hold for as long as you want, applying gentle pressure with the thumb. You can do this with either hand.

---

18 April

Honestly, how often do you really savour your food, truly appreciating the taste? Connect with your sense of taste with this flavoursome meditation practice.

You'll need something that packs a lot of flavour, such as a square of chocolate (the darker the better – maybe a nice piece of Easter egg!) or a raisin. Settle yourself in a comfortable position, with your tasty morsel. Take time to look at it – the size, the colour, the shape. Now smell it. Take in the different aromas. Enjoy taking your time to savour everything about it. Now place it in your mouth. Don't chew it just yet! Become aware of how it alights your taste buds. Slowly start to chew. Keep chewing. Notice the textures, the depth of the flavours. Really chewing, only swallow when it's totally broken down. Be curious. Do you still enjoy the flavour? Has it become too intense? When we practise meditation like this, with focus on the sense of taste, it also helps us to cultivate another type of taste, the quality of discernment, helping us to make good choices in life.

19 April

I love my feet – and I tell them regularly! They've supported my body for many years and many miles, with hardly any complaint...not even when I squeeze them into my favourite party shoes.

Take off your shoes and socks today and look at your feet. Consider all the muscles and bones that make them up – truly amazing! Stand on the earth (even better if you can do this outside). Wriggle your toes. Spread them out before placing them back down on the earth. Can you lift the big toe of each foot, pressing the other four toes into the earth? How about pushing the big toe down whilst you lift the other four? Roll the weight inwards and then outwards a few times. Now rock forwards and backwards. Lift onto the balls of your feet without letting your ankles fall in or your weight roll to the outside of the foot. Finally, come to a still point, feeling the weight settle across the ball of the foot and the centre of the heel. Just beautiful! This is both calming and helps to strengthen your feet.

---

20 April

Sitting on your heels isn't always an easy thing to do, but the benefits that come from sitting in this position might make you think it's worth a try. It helps to calm and settle the body, in my experience, and can be particularly helpful if you lack belief in yourself. The position of the feet brings flexibility to the ankles, as well as strengthening the arches of your feet, which has a positive knock-on effect on the health of your back. It's also good for your digestive system, encouraging the smooth passage of food through the gut.

Come to kneeling, sitting on your heels, with your big toes together so the heels relax out a little. Sit in the "cup" you make with your feet (your cup may runneth over, which is absolutely fine). Lengthen your tailbone towards the floor, so that you are drawing in gently the flesh away from your pants and taking out the nip of an exaggerated arch in the lower back. Make it more comfortable if you need to, experimenting with rolled up blankets under the ankles, under the knees, between the thighs, between your bottom and your heels. Let your spine lengthen and your breath deepen as you relax into this understated posture. Hold for a few breaths if you can.

21 April

Getting out in the morning light is super beneficial, and a lovely thing to do in spring. Twenty minutes' exposure to morning light can slow the onset of common age-related challenges such as insomnia, cognitive impairment and depression. Blue spectrum light is at its bluest in a morning, helping to keep our circadian rhythm in harmony. Our circadian rhythm is what sets our body clock and governs the timing of cortisol (to keep us awake and aware during the day) and melatonin (so we can sleep at night). Furthermore, as we age, our pupils narrow and the lenses of our eyes become less efficient, so we take in less blue spectrum light, throwing out the circadian rhythm and leading to the problems mentioned, as well as being linked to an increase in the risk of insulin resistance, heart disease and cancers, as the circadian rhythm affects key hormonal processes. Lots of reasons then to get out in these hopefully longer, lighter, milder days.

22 April

The food we eat can have a big effect on our ability to concentrate. If you need to focus or are struggling to stop your mind wandering, it's worth knowing that high-sugar diets, also low and no-carb diets, have been shown to have a negative impact on thinking. Better to opt for healthy carbs, such as wholemeal bread, brown rice and sweet potatoes.

Here are some other great brain foods:

- Berries, red grapes and plums – full of epicatechin, a powerful antioxidant that protects the brain's neurons.
- Salmon, sardines, avocados, nuts and seeds – for your essential fatty acids, low levels of which have been linked to memory loss.

- Cauliflower – contains citicoline to improve the long-term memory function in the frontal lobe of the brain.
- Eggs, chicken, fish and beans – rich in choline, which has been shown to reduce the brain changes associated with dementia.

---

23 April

I have another fabulous variation of the "cat posture" today. This one, I find soothing for the lower back, particularly for easing sore sacroiliac joints.

Start on all fours, with hands under shoulders, and knees under hips. Your spine is in its natural position. Gently draw the flesh away from your pants to give you some support. Allow your weight to shift slightly forwards, towards your hands. Then shift your weight backwards, towards your hips. Flow, steadily, between these two movements, keeping your spine in a neutral position, parallel to the floor throughout, so that you are not moving too far in either direction. Allow your spine to lengthen with each movement.

From the same starting position, now make a circle in one direction with your hips. It should feel comfortable and soothing, keeping your spine parallel to the floor. After a few rounds in one direction, circle your hips in the opposite direction. Finish these moves by stretching back, lowering your bottom to your heels, before uncurling into sitting.

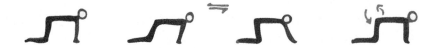

24 April

Staying hydrated is such an easy way to keep your body on your side.

Here are a few things dehydration can cause:

- Headaches
- Digestive problems
- Back pain.

Good hydration gives support to our immune system (see 8 February). Perhaps a more surprising benefit to staying hydrated is that it can help lower raised cholesterol levels. Our body stores water in fat, so if we are not drinking enough, the body will store fat to hold onto the fluid it has.

Making sure you drink enough can also help your mental health. If you are frequently dehydrated, it can cause the body stress – the body thinks it doesn't have enough to drink, leading to symptoms of anxiety.

I've always found warm water to be more hydrating than cold – sipped rather than gulped. Your urine needs to be pale and odourless. If it's dark with a strong odour, then drink a bit more. If it is completely clear, you might just want to ease up a little on the water, as it is possible to drink too much.

---

25 April

There are times when we all commit crimes against wisdom! By this, I am referring to the times when we do something that we really know will not benefit us, or indeed we don't do something that we know full well will help us if we do. For example, speaking negatively about ourselves, eating something we know will not suit us, not getting enough sleep because we've been up late scrolling through our social media feeds. Today, I ask you just to be open to this thought, to consider areas of your life where you might be committing a crime against your inner wisdom. If you feel like it, delve a little deeper. Why do you do this? What is the pay off? Is it a habit? Do you feel you don't deserve self-care? Is this something you feel ready to explore?

Self-care is essential and is never selfish. Fight crimes against wisdom by making regular, small tweaks to your lifestyle. Stick at these tweaks, commit to them for 21 days (see 10 February) and notice how making wise choices becomes second nature.

---

26 April

I hope you enjoy this kitchari recipe, a favourite of mine in spring. This is my take on a meal I first had many years ago at the Dru Yoga centre (if you like this, check out Keith Squires' book, *Cooking with Love*). It helps to take dampness out of the body, as well as being warm and nourishing, plus it's packed full of anti-inflammatory spices. This serves four people.

- Soak 100g of mung beans overnight. Rinse and add to a big pan with 100g of rinsed brown rice. Gently simmer in vegetable stock for about 30 minutes. Start with about 250ml, adding more as needed.
- Add one thinly chopped leek, one diced carrot, one chopped celery stick and a diced potato. Cook for another 20 minutes. Add more water/stock, if needed.
- In a small saucepan with a tight lid, melt a tablespoon of ghee. Add half a teaspoon each of cumin seeds and black mustard seeds. Put the lid on and wait until you hear it popping.
- Remove from the heat. Add one red onion, chopped finely, and about a 2cm piece of grated fresh ginger, along with half a teaspoon each of ground cumin, turmeric and coriander. If you have it, you can also add a pinch of asafoetida (also known as "hing"). Be careful when you remove the lid of the pan, as the hot mustard seeds spit! Return to the heat, with the lid off, and gently fry, stirring to stop it sticking until the onion is soft.
- Add the spice mixture to the big pan of mung beans, rice and vegetables. Add the juice of either half a lemon or half a lime. You also need a bit of sweet – traditionally, Indian sugar called "jaggery" would be used, but I like to add a tablespoon of desiccated coconut.
- Mix it all in. Serve with chopped fresh coriander on top. It is lovely with basmati rice and steamed green veggies!

27 April

Once you get used to allowing your physical body to relax (see 4 January), you might like to add in an extra layer of relaxation, allowing for a deeper experience.

After the squeeze and release stage of your relaxation, let your awareness return to your feet. Visualise that you are bringing light into each part of your body, each time you breathe in, working from the feet up. As you exhale, let the light relax that part of your body, feeling it soften and release. Draw the light all the way up your legs and around your hips. Let the light flow up the spine, radiating out into the muscles of the back. Feel it in your abdomen, softening the digestive organs, into the ribs, chest, heart and lungs. Light flows in through the hands all the way up the arms to the shoulders, around the neck, over the face and head. Spend the last few moments of your relaxation bathing in the light that fills every cell of your body. Healing and rejuvenating. Feel yourself as a body of light.

---

28 April

Earlier in the year, we touched on the sense of smell (see 7 February) and how this sense accesses the limbic system of our brain, an area that controls emotion, so it's no surprise that a scent has the power to trigger a memory. Why not explore aromatherapy a bit further? Connect with the healing properties of smell and discover its power to help us find peace and calm. I love to put a couple of drops of my favourite essential oil on a hanky, so I can waft it under my nose when I need to settle, changing the scent as required. Here are a couple of my favourites:

- For focus and clarity – frankincense, rosemary.
- To energise – peppermint, grapefruit.
- To soothe and relax – rose, sweet orange.

Always remember to check if an essential oil is safe for you to use.

29 April

Counting breath is a useful technique to learn to help you feel more in control - it gives the mind something to do instead of causing mischief! Start by sitting comfortably, allowing your breath to settle. Maybe you can feel it deepen. Find a steady rhythm. Breathe in and out through the nose, if possible.

Once established, and you are happy (let this take as long as it takes - minutes, days, weeks...there's no hurry), start to equalise the in and the out-breaths (keep breathing relaxed, never forced, and if it feels uncomfortable in any way, then stop). Aim to inhale for a count of four, and exhale for a count of four. Continue with this rhythm, breathing in and out through the nose for a few minutes if it feels right for you. When you are ready to finish, take a couple of deeper breaths before moving your body and returning to your day, peaceful and refreshed.

---

30 April

Meditation is so much more than a means to an end. It goes beyond relaxation and it's more than simple concentration. It's about **being**, without judgement. For me, one of the greatest gifts meditation gives is acceptance. Sit quietly and practise coming into harmony with all that is. Accept the environment you are in. Accept your body as it is. Accept the mind, with all its chatter, as this will never stop altogether - thinking and chattering are the mind's job. Accept all with love, joy and compassion, without judgement or the need to change anything (I appreciate this is easier said than done!). Acceptance will help you to move more readily into a meditative state, and as you practise more and more, you will find that the power of acceptance radiates out into all aspects of your life.

May

1 May

Hopefully, the weather is warming up by now, with the sun shining. The birds are singing, colour is blossoming out all over – it is truly a season of positive, creative energy. The lyrical, spiritual writer, Kahlil Gibran, advises us to "be like a flower and turn your face to the sun". Taking adequate sun protection precautions, of course, why not do this today? Not only will you feel a lift emotionally, but you'll also soak up a little vitamin D if you're outside, to lift your physical body. Either sit outside or inside, in a sunny ray, settle yourself, and turn your face up towards the sun. Each inhalation is a gift. Breathe in prana, the very essence of life.

2 May

Let's make the most of the lighter mornings and the rising energy of May with this empowering walking and breathing practice. It was taught to me many years ago, and whilst I don't use it all the time, when I do, I am always amazed by how uplifted I feel after. It's my go-to practice if I feel in need of a shot of enthusiasm, vitality or self-confidence.

You just need 15 minutes to get out for a walk. Start off at a brisk pace to give your circulation a boost. Breathing deeply, but naturally and comfortably, inhale, then as you exhale, touch the tips of your fingers with the thumb, each one in turn from the index to the little finger (one exhalation for all four fingers). At the end of each exhalation, shout/say/whisper/internalise (delete as applicable) the word **"yes"**. Continue this practice until the end of your walk, if you can. By the end, I hope you are feeling energised and filled with positivity. This is most effective if done first thing in a morning before the busyness of the day has time to intrude, but this is not always possible, so practise when you need it.

3 May

Staying with the overall feeling of positivity and happiness, today, I have a powerful quote from Gandhi for you to consider.

"Happiness is when what you think, what you say and what you do are in harmony."

Can you relate to this? It has been my experience that if our words, actions and intentions are not aligned, we create a sense of duality, we are not living our truth, which only ever seems to lead to upset and confusion. Spring is a good time to reassess our thoughts and actions, ensuring we are being true to ourselves.

---

4 May

Our ability to balance often deteriorates as we get older, but it doesn't have to be this way. Think of your balance function like a muscle - the more you use it, the stronger it gets. How we balance depends a lot on the strength and flexibility of our feet and ankles. This simple exercise works on improving both. Sit or stand, in bare feet, with a towel in front of your feet. Use your toes to grab hold of the towel. Use your toes to draw the towel towards you before releasing your grip. Repeat as often as you want.

---

5 May

Research shows that looking at water can lift our mood. Maybe there's a deep meaning as to why this should be - because we are 60% water - or perhaps it reminds us of our nurturing gestation period in amniotic fluid. Or maybe it's simply because it puts us in mind of summer holidays and relaxation. Whatever the reason, if you are, or can be, near water - a river, the sea, a lake or a stream - what luck! Spend some time there being soothed by the flow and rhythm of the water. Listen to the sounds and immerse yourself in the colours, shapes and patterns. If not, get creative. Add a water feature to your garden, or a bird bath. Perhaps you could fill a beautiful bowl with water and place it near your workstation or on a window ledge, with the added bonus of filling the space with beneficial negative ions. Occasionally, let your gaze settle on the water, allowing yourself to become calm and tranquil.

6 May

I hope you've had chance to try out some of the seasonal tips I've woven through the months of spring. As mentioned at the beginning of the season, spring is a transitional season, the bridge between winter and summer, and as we approach the final stage of this transition, I would like to consider the yoga concept of "sukha". Sukha loosely translates to "ease" or "sweet", or sometimes it is translated as "good space".

Finding space is important at any time, but especially so in spring, as it helps our vital force (prana) to move freely around our body. Otherwise, it might get caught in the stagnation of winter, in the constricted areas of the body.

All the lifestyle tips I have shared have helped us to move into a space of sukha.

- Follow the seasonal foodie tips.
- Move your body in ways that release stagnation from the hips and legs, typically the heaviest parts of our body. Consider adding squatting movements into your day – these are just the job for improving the flow of prana!
- Conserve your vital energy and avoid stress and tension where you can.
- Use your breath to create space where you feel there is tightness or constriction. Literally direct prana (life force) to where you need it most.

---

7 May

We are well into hay-fever season, which can be a miserable time for many. Here is one of my mainstay mudras for this time. "Bhramara" mudra is good for autoimmune disorders, especially allergies and respiratory disorders.

On each hand, curl the index finger into the root of the thumb, then lightly connect the tip of the thumb to the inside of the top of the middle finger. The ring and little finger extend. Keep the hands relaxed, resting on your knees, as you hold this mudra, breathing naturally. Hopefully you will find it relaxes and deepens your breath, making breathing much easier.

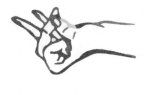

---

8 May

Do you find yourself easily distracted? I know I do! One tip that has helped me to become more productive, with the knock-on effect of feeling less overwhelmed, is to focus on one task at a time. Multi-tasking is unproductive and inefficient, regardless of what your busy mind is telling you. When you pick up a task, focus only on this one task. Complete what you need to do with it, then consciously put it down before moving onto the next task. I find it even more effective if I consciously set that task down when completed, and then either move my body or do some breathing before I move on, drawing a line between tasks. At the start of a new job, I use the affirmation "I am picking this task up" and at the end I affirm "I am putting this task down". Don't keep all your tasks juggling. Chances are you'll never finish everything, and it's a waste of time and energy.

---

9 May

How we start our day does make a difference. The first hour of the day has been revered by yogis for centuries as a time for building prana (life force) with yoga, pranayama (breathing techniques) and meditation, providing time to check in with ourselves.

If the minute you wake up you are checking your phone or planning your day, chances are the day will carry on in this busy way. Start your day with some quiet time, to check in with yourself, and you might just find your day runs a little smoother. I like to light a candle as I practise my morning yoga and meditation, the flame providing a focus for peace and stillness.

10 May

There are two things I consider essential and that I check in with every day.

The first is myself, first job when I wake up. How do I feel? What do I need to do today to feel even better? What do I want to achieve today? I find it useful to have a plan for the day ahead, so that the day doesn't run away with me.

I also check in with myself at regular intervals throughout the day. Am I holding onto any tension or is there constriction in any part of my body? How are my energy levels? Do I need to laugh a bit more, or lighten up? And, ultimately, what can I do to make myself a bit more comfortable?

The second thing I check in with is the natural world. This connection gives me the opportunity to absorb the energy of the elements and enjoy a moment of calm, providing me with a little extra vitality and clarity.

---

11 May

We all have days when we just don't feel ourselves. Try this fantastic move for lifting your energy, clearing your auric field (particularly useful if you've been with a "mood hoover") and bringing movement into your whole body.

Hold your hands by your heart centre, as if you are holding a ball, taking a moment to focus on the space between your hands. If you like visualisation, you might like to see this as a ball of light. Keeping your awareness with this ball of energy and its size and shape, move it up towards your right shoulder, then down towards your right ribs, now take it diagonally across the midline of your body to your left shoulder, down towards the left lower ribcage, before coming diagonally past the heart centre up to your right shoulder. Keep this movement flowing in this sideways on figure of eight, like the sign of infinity. Once you get into the rhythm, maintaining your awareness of the ball, you can explore moving in different ways.

- Keep it flowing around your thoracic region to release tension from the neck and shoulders.
- Take the movement higher, overhead if it's OK for you, to give yourself a great stretch, perfect if you've been hunched over a screen all day.

- To lift your mood, try moving the ball of light in a big, wide, sweeping movement to each side.
- Take your legs wide, shifting your weight from side to side – this is great for working the hips and legs.
- If my back is feeling tight, I like to do the figure-of-eight movement from a forward bend, with my feet wider.
- Another great position to ease a tight lower back is to keep the flow going whilst in an easy squat.

Be creative, listen to your body, move mindfully, and go with the flow.

---

12 May

The "crocodile" is a useful yoga posture to add into your repertoire. Use it when you are feeling overwrought and unsettled emotionally. Use it to help you feel calm, relaxed and grounded. It's also effective for relieving a griping tummy, stomach upsets and symptoms of IBS.

Lie on your front, preferably on the floor, but you can do it on your bed if it's better for you. Fold your elbows so that you can rest your forehead on the backs of your hands. Walk your feet and legs out, to a comfortable distance. Allow your heels to fall in and your toes to point outwards (rest your ankles/feet on a roll of blanket if you need extra cushioning or support).

Take a few breaths here, feeling the connection you make with the earth. Now take your awareness to your shoulder girdle. Use your out-breath to relax tension from the shoulders. Do the same with your pelvic girdle, relaxing the hips and legs on the exhalation. Now imagine the back being nourished as your in-breath travels the full length of your spine, the relaxation radiating out to all the muscles of your torso as you breathe out.

Rest here for as long as you feel you need to.

---

13 May

It's so important to keep our feet moving, in all different ways, to keep the muscles strong, the joints flexible and to stop the fascia from become tight and sticky. We've explored a few movements already this year, so I hope you are noticing that your feet are more responsive to your connection with the earth and that you've noticed how this benefits all your other joints and helps you to move with greater ease.

Today, I invite you to pay more attention to your feet and, in particular, the toes. Spread out all your toes and wriggle them. Now see if you can fit your fingers between your toes (your index finger between your big and second toe, your middle finger between the second and third toes, etc) on both feet. Do they fit, or do you need to open your toes out? Can you rest for a few breaths with your fingers between your toes?

Now remove your fingers, give your toes another wriggle, and massage each of the toe joints. Creep your thumb up and down the inner part of the toes, massaging the spaces between them, to help them spread out. I bet your toes feel all tingly and warm, and much more flexible, when you've finished.

---

14 May

You've probably realised by now how important I think sleep and relaxation are, which leads me nicely into one of my favourite breathing techniques - alternate nostril breathing. It is the perfect breath for bringing calm and emotional balance, and increasing vitality, as it reduces stress and anxiety levels, helping the mind to settle.

Sit comfortably. Rest the middle finger of your right hand on the bridge of your nose, close the right nostril with your thumb and inhale through the left nostril. Close the left nostril with your ring or little finger as you release your thumb from the right nostril, so that you can exhale through your right nostril. Keeping the fingers where they are, inhale through the right nostril. Exhale through the left nostril, as you close the right with your thumb. This is one round. Continue in this way, alternating between the nostrils, building up to 10 rounds, assuming it feels comfortable. Stop altogether if you feel lightheaded. There should never be pain or discomfort – breathing should always feel relaxed, never forced.

If you are unable to breathe through your nostrils, then visualise the breath moving between the nostrils – it works just as well.

---

15 May

Summer is just around the corner. As we welcome the "flower moon", we celebrate life – let the good times roll!

Connect with the glorious, creative energy of May's full moon by filling your life with flowers. Get out in your garden, or any green space where you can look at the splendid floral display that Mother Nature gifts us in May. Take time to properly look at the beauty of the flowers, smell them, watch how life springs up all around them. Be still here amongst the flowers.

How else can you bring flowers into your day? Of course, you might want to display some fresh flowers or a flowering plant. Maybe you could be a bit more creative. Press some flowers, use them to make greetings cards. Lose yourself in botanical artwork. Make perfume (did you do this as a child?) or spritz your favourite flowery perfume or essential oil. Make some potpourri. Use edible petals in your cooking or try a cooling drink of rose tea. Whatever you do, make sure it's a pleasure.

You might well have picked up that the flower moon is all about abundance, pleasure, fun and laughter. If you like writing in your journal, consider how these qualities manifest in your life and, more importantly, how you can increase them!

16 May

Where there is pain, there will usually be constriction. Help to soften a painful area with some vibration therapy.

Move yourself into a comfortable position and allow your breath to settle. Start to hum gently as you exhale, feeling the breath moving in your throat and through the lips. Relax into the practice. Once you have established a steady breathing rhythm, direct the out-breath, and with it hum to the part of your body that needs additional healing energy. Feel the vibrations building. As they do, feel the tissues of your body softening and releasing. You might find the area feels locked at first but keep going (this may take a few separate relaxations, no need to rush). Eventually, you will feel the vibrations spreading outwards as the constriction releases, allowing the free flow of energy. You can practise this if you don't have pain. Just allow the vibrations to flow throughout your body, for a deeply nourishing relaxation.

---

17 May

Oh, the misery of hay fever! Here are six of the most useful things I've found for bringing calm to an overactive autoimmune system and dampening-down spring and summer allergies.

- Make sure you get plenty of relaxation and rest – I've never met anyone with an overactive autoimmune system that isn't tired on a very deep level.
- Practise the following breathing flow – 10 deep yogic breaths (see 31 March), 10 alternate nostril breaths (see 14 May) and five humming bee breaths (see 16 June).
- Cut down on mucus-forming food – sugar, dairy, wheat.
- Try saltwater nasal washing (see 4 March), particularly after you've been outside. It helps to keep sinuses clear and flushes away pollen.
- Place a little coconut oil or shea butter in your nostrils to act as a barrier against pollen spores when you go out.
- Consider taking turmeric.

18 May

Sometimes, when your back is aching (maybe you've been sat too long or been bent over too much), you know you need a good stretch out. This is one of my favourites, gentle and supportive enough to do when my back is sore, yet still giving that much-needed length through my spine.

Start on all fours in the classic "cat posture" (see 19 February). You might want to practise some of the cat stretches you now know before moving onto the next stretch. Place your hands just a little bit forwards of your shoulders (further, if you are long in back or don't feel a satisfying stretch), with middle fingers, if they will, pointing the way forwards. Push down into the tips of all your fingers, so that they do not lift from the earth, as you lower your bottom towards your heels. Place a cushion between your heels and your bottom if you don't comfortably reach. Spend a little time here and relax your hips and bottom towards your feet – this should give you a beautiful stretch. Don't force it. Then take a couple of breaths, fully relaxed in this "extended child" position, sliding your hands and arms further forwards if it feels good. To come out, walk your hands back to your shoulders, and slowly push up into kneeling.

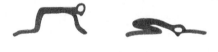

---

19 May

Try the breath for self-empowerment today, a staple of Dru Yoga practice. Use it when you need a boost to your confidence, vitality or enthusiasm.

Best done from standing (see the "mountain pose" on 9 January), bring your arms in front of you, crossed at the wrists. Inhale as you draw your crossed hands up and overhead, leading with your elbows so that you can keep your shoulders relaxed. At the top, let the arms separate, exhaling as they float down to your sides, bending the knees as you go. Bring the arms back in front of you, crossed at the wrists, alternating which arm is in front. As you inhale and take the arms up and over, straighten the legs. Coordinate all your movements with the breath. Feel your spine lengthen and expand, your chest area opening as you breathe in, releasing tension as you breathe out.

Repeat this breath as many times as you feel necessary. You can make it stronger by moving the feet wider apart, deeply bending the knees as you exhale. This version helps you to feel grounded as you become aware of the strength of your legs.

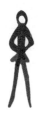 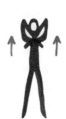 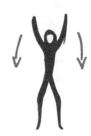

---

20 May

In this month of rising energy, hopefully you are also finding your own energy levels are rising. This is a time to be creative and dynamic. Tap into that solar energy by connecting with your fire centre, the "manipura" chakra, situated in the area of your navel. As the sun shines out, energising the planets of our solar system, let the energy of manipura radiate out, filling you with vitality.

- Like attracts like. If you want to be creative, then get busy being creative – just make a start. If you want to raise your energy levels, lift your mood and feel more dynamic, it often helps to get moving...dynamically! Dancing is a fabulous way to experience vitality, in my opinion.
- In your journal, consider your energy levels. What/who depletes your energy? What/who have you noticed lifts your energy? Do you waste your own energy getting angry? What would you do if you had plenty of energy? Looking at your musings, are there any changes you could make?
- Follow the wisdom of our furry friends – find yourself a sunray to lie in for your relaxation time. If you are outside, make sure you are not going to burn! If there is no sun, imagine it. Whatever your sun relaxation, allow its warmth and radiance to fill every cell of your body, rejuvenating and energising.

- For a shot of dynamism or to tap into your creative well, wear bright yellow and bring it into your environment. Let sunflowers and buttercups be your colour inspiration.
- Glorious topaz is a gemstone to help you connect with manipura, whilst citrine brings balance.
- If it's OK for you to use, add a drop of ginger or lemongrass essential oil to your bathwater or in a body cream that you can massage into your body, especially around your abdomen. These oils will help to relax a griping tummy and soothe your digestive system, as well as drying up any dampness that might be putting out your digestive fire.
- Practise some of the lying and standing twisting movements that I'm sharing through the months.

---

21 May

Stomach upsets often make an appearance in late spring and summer – it's all that extra heat in the digestive system as the "pitta" dosha rises. This is exacerbated as we head towards holiday season, travelling to new places, eating and drinking things that our body is not used to.

In Ayurveda, our digestive fire is known as "agni", and keeping our digestive fires well stoked without allowing them to rage out of control is a primary concern. Throughout the year, I am sharing tips and ideas to help smooth the path of digestion (which I trust have been helping) so that your body is best able to digest and utilise the food you eat. I find it particularly useful to support my gut at this time of year with "triphala", perhaps the most common of Ayurvedic supplements. Mildly laxative (non-addictive) it helps regulate the flow of food through your intestines, as well as bringing balance to your appetite. Hoovering up toxins and nourishing your gut, it supports your digestive system on every level. It's long been a staple in my diet, and I always take a little bit more around holidays to make sure that my digestion stays in tip-top condition.

22 May

If you've been following this book from the beginning of the year, I'm hoping you have been inspired to practise meditation, which probably means you've started to buffer against a few challenges! This is good, it shows that energy is shifting. As a meditation teacher, one of the questions I get asked most frequently is "Why do I find it difficult to meditate at home?" Let me start by saying that this is both a common and a normal experience of meditation. Put simply, there are far more distractions at home than there are in a dedicated meditation class. You are more likely to be distracted by other people if you are at home – it's not always possible to shut people out, or you forget to put your phone on silent, or the window cleaner arrives. Plus, your mind has a very easy time of distracting you when you are at home. Does this inner dialogue sound familiar? "Sitting in silence? Have you seen that pile of ironing? I could be using this spare time to catch up with jobs. I wonder what's on the TV?" And so, it goes on. Meditating at home is fantastic, but it does require more discipline, which can be tricky if you are not yet into a silent sitting routine.

My advice is don't lose heart, stick with it. Get into a routine if you can. Try different meditation techniques (there are many in this book, and many more besides), for a few weeks at least – this gives you plenty of time to learn and get comfortable with the practice. Jumping from practice to practice is often another trick of the mind, convincing you there is a better meditation available.

If you've just picked up this book, then maybe today is the day you try some silent sitting. No expectation, just be still and silent for a few moments. We all have to start somewhere.

---

23 May

I first came across the dazzling healing powers of turmeric several years ago when I was struggling with a serious autoimmune condition. Packed with cell-protecting flavonoids, turmeric is often referred to as nature's steroid for its anti-inflammatory properties, used in Ayurvedic medicine to soothe aching joints and support various bodily systems, including the digestive organs, brain, heart and skin (applied as a paste, it's also great for boils, wounds and sores, in my experience, though do make sure to cover the turmeric paste as it's terrible for turning everything it touches, yellow!). It's also been shown to be a useful ally in the fight against age-related diseases. A common culinary spice, turmeric is best taken with other food, in particular black pepper. You can even add it to warm milk for a tasty, rejuvenating drink.

---

24 May

I hope you are enjoying and, indeed, benefitting from all the moves we are practising for keeping the spine mobile and pain-free. This gentle flow of stretches for the back promotes good spinal health, including a great movement for strengthening the anti-hump muscles. You may have noticed this "hump" at the back of the neck/top of the shoulders, appearing in older people, so this move also keeps our spine youthful.

Avoid these moves if your back muscles are in spasm, you have an overactive thyroid gland, a hiatus hernia, a peptic ulcer or have had recent abdominal surgery.

- Lie on the floor (on a yoga mat for comfort if you have one), on your front, with your forehead on the mat. Legs comfortably together, ankles relaxed.
- Stretch your arms along the floor in front of you, resting on the floor, so that you are in a long line. Inhale, stretching into your fingers and your toes. Relax. Repeat again, this time tucking the toes under, stretching into the fingers and the heels, and relax.
- Bring your hands either side of your head, with your thumbs in line with your eyes. Draw the flesh away from your pants, gently taking the arch out of the small of your back, lengthening your tailbone. As you breath in, lengthen your spine, lifting your head, shoulders and chest. Draw your elbows in so you can rest on your forearms, like a sphinx. Take a couple of breaths here, lengthening your spine, with your sternum moving forwards. Can you relax your buttock muscles?
- If it feels comfortable, as you breathe out, turn your head to one side, looking over the shoulder. Breathe in as you bring your head back to look forwards. Breathe out. Turn to the other side, breathe in, and return your head to the centre. Repeat three times, feeling a subtle, nurturing squeeze along the length of the spine.
- From the central position, still resting on your forearms, allow your head to relax forwards, with your chin towards the chest. Pause here, allowing your neck to relax, totally supported by your arms. Now lift the head by stacking

the neck vertebrae one on top of the other, by drawing the chin in as you lift the head. Be aware not to jut the chin up and take care not to strain. When your head is lifted, your chin should be parallel to the floor and you should be looking forwards. Hopefully, you can feel the muscles at the back of your neck engaging as you lift the head. Repeat twice more if you are happy to.

- To come out, lift the elbows a little and move them outwards, so you can lower to the earth.
- Bring your hands closer to your waist, push yourself up onto all fours, then lower your bottom to your heels to release your back. Stay here for a couple of breaths, either with the arms outstretched or having brought them in closer, before uncurling into kneeling.

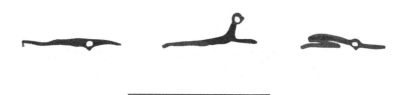

---

25 May

Here's a delightful practice to soothe, relax and refresh, and it takes just a couple of minutes. It's particularly nice to do if you need a break from looking at the computer screen.

- With clean hands, rub the palms together until they become nice and warm.
- Close your eyes and place your warmed palms over your closed eyes. Feel the warmth of your hands soothing your eyelids, radiating outwards, bringing a sense of peace and relaxation.
- Still with your hands over your eyes, open your eyes, into the darkness of your palms. Again, let your eyes bathe in the warmth.
- Start to lower the hands, allowing chinks of light in, and gently massage your face and neck.

26 May

Have you ever spent time with someone and left feeling somewhat drained of energy, or perhaps in a mood and you can't tell where it has come from? I think we all know a mood hoover! There are many ways to protect and clear our energy when we've been with such a person. Here are six of my favourites:

- When with someone you know drains your energy, stand or sit with your toes turned inwards slightly, place your hands over your navel area and try to avoid direct eye contact. This protects our energy centres. Strange, I know, but I always find it effective.
- Assuming you are OK to use essential oils, you could try one of the following. In my experience, people respond differently to different oils, so if one doesn't work, then try another.
    - Place a spot of vetivert (to read more about this essential oil, see 11 November) at the base of your spine.
    - Put a spot of juniper on each wrist, then move it all around your body, starting with your feet, working up by criss-crossing the arms front and back.
    - Using a spot of calming oil such as chamomile on one finger, place it on your abdomen, about three fingers' width down from your navel, circling your finger in an anticlockwise direction, slowly and in a small area.
- There are many crystals and gemstones said to protect energy, transforming negative energy into positive. Why not explore the ones that feel good for you? My personal favourites are hematite and rose quartz.
- After your meeting, clear your aura with a cold shower, or at least splash your face with cold water and flick it around yourself.
- Get outside. It is even better if you have chance to go for a brisk walk.
- Hold your hands at the heart centre, as if holding a football. Move the hands in a figure-of-eight movement on its side (see 11 May for more details). Make the movement large and sweeping, taking it wide and large to each side, always crossing in front of the heart. This helps to clear negativity from your aura, so is of particular use if you leave your meeting in a mood you were not previously aware of.

27 May

As the weather starts to warm up, you may well find yourself becoming increasingly tetchy. Calm any irritation and help yourself to re-balance with this beautiful twist.

From standing, allow yourself to fold into a comfortable forward bend, walking your feet out a couple of shoulder-widths apart, knees soft, hands resting on the floor (or rest your hands either on a chair or on blocks to raise you up a bit, if it feels like too much of a stretch). If you are not comfortable here, or there is any reason why you don't want the pressure in your head (due to cataracts, glaucoma, weak eye capillaries or blood pressure problems), then you can do the same move from sitting on a chair with your hands resting on the seat.

Press your left hand into the earth (or whatever you are resting on), drawing your right hand up, across the chest, keeping your elbow bent. This will facilitate a delicious rotation in your spine, your right ribcage rotating towards the ceiling. If it feels comfortable, straighten the right arm, with fingers pointing up towards the ceiling. You might want to straighten your legs but keep the connection of your left hand with the earth. Here you are in perfect alignment between the heavens and the earth. Bending your elbow, fold your right arm in, with your hand back to the earth, softening your knees once more. Now do the movement with the left arm, rotating your ribs and extending your arm up on the inhalation, relaxing back towards the earth with the exhalation. Repeat three times on each side. Walk your feet back to the centre, bend your knees and slowly uncurl into standing. You might like to spend a few minutes in the "crocodile posture" to really allow yourself to be still.

Hopefully, you feel a little more zen-like, as this movement shifts stuck energy from the lower centre (where all the egotistical, emotional stuff lurks) up to the heart centre for transformation into something more positive.

28 May

Bring a little calm to any moment with this simple awareness exercise. It's also a lovely way to settle yourself before a meditation practice.

Sitting or standing comfortably, become aware of the length of your spine, as you feel your breath settle. Take your focus to the base of your spine. As you breathe in, let your awareness travel all the way up your spine, at the back of your body, to the crown of your head – note how much of your spine you are aware of. Are there any gaps? Do you find it a challenge to get all the way to the top? As you breathe out, your awareness moves from the crown of the head down the front of your body, to the base, following the shape of the spine, again with awareness. Repeat this circle three times.

Your experience of this may well be different every time. There's no need to judge, just be the witness. Whatever your experience, hopefully it will bring you a few moments of tranquillity.

---

29 May

We've thought quite a bit about how to start our days, so let's not forget some beautiful night-time rituals. Before bed, put aside 10–15 minutes to massage your feet, head and hands. Start by resting your hands on your feet, and stroke them. Let your thumbs and fingers work into the muscles and joints. With clean hands, rest your hands on your head. Gently pull your hair, then imagine you are washing your hair, working into your scalp. Finish by working some nourishing cream into your hands, fingers and wrists. You might like to add in a facial massage, spending extra time smoothing in your face cream. Repeating this massage routine every night is a signal to your body that you are letting go of the day, and now it's time for sleep.

---

30 May

Yesterday, I mentioned how beneficial you might find a scalp massage before bed. Exploring this a little further, scalp massages have been used for thousands of years in Asia. You might have experienced a delightful Indian head massage, which cares for the scalp and improves circulation to the hair roots which, in turn, promotes lustrous, healthy hair. Scalp massages are also used to alleviate headaches, release stress and tension, and aid a good night's sleep.

Pour a couple of teaspoons of coconut or sesame oil into a dish. Take up a little with your fingers and warm it in your hands, then apply to your scalp, starting at the crown, sliding your fingers downwards and outwards from this point. The aim is to get the oil onto the scalp, not to oil the hair. Take your hands to your hairline and work back towards the base of your skull, making small circles with your fingertips. Make sure you move gently and steadily around the scalp – being too rough or moving quickly can damage the roots of your hair. Treat every part of your body with kindness and respect.

Use an old pillowcase on your pillow when you go to bed, in case some of the oil transfers onto the pillowcase as you sleep. In the morning, wash your hair with a light shampoo. If you prefer to wash the oil out before bed, give it at least 15 minutes to soak into your scalp before shampooing.

---

31 May

I do enjoy a crunchy, savoury snack. Yes, I'm talking crisps and peanuts! Looking for a tasty, more health-conscious alternative, I happened upon seeds toasted with tamari (Japanese wheat-free soy sauce), and I absolutely love them. The tamari gives that savoury hit of umami, the crunch and taste come from the toasted seeds and, best of all, I get all the health benefits too! Seeds are a great source of anti-ageing nutrients such as Omega-3 fats and antioxidants, along with nervous system-supporting vitamin B.

I put a good handful of sunflower, pumpkin and flax (linseed) seeds into a dry frying pan. I let them toast a few seconds on a low heat before adding a good slosh of tamari, about a tablespoon. Experiment to get the taste right for you – too much and the seeds lose their crunch and I find them a bit salty, but you want enough to get the umami kick. Mix the seeds in with the tamari so that they are all coated, and continue to fry them. Keep stirring to get an even toast. I remove from the heat when I hear the seeds start to pop. Let them cool, mixing them up regularly to stop them sticking together. Store in an airtight container once completely cooled. Add them to your morning porridge, sprinkle them over soups and salads, or just eat them!

June

1 June

Have you felt the energy of the season change? We are moving into summer, being naturally ushered into a new way of living. Let's start and end today by welcoming in the new season.

In the summer months, you might naturally find yourself waking up earlier. Go with it and start your day with some calm and quiet before the busyness of the world begins. This will be even more soothing if you are able to get outside for an alfresco yoga practice, a gentle stroll, or some quiet time listening to the birds.

End your day peacefully if you can, with a still reflection of your day and some slow, deep breathing. It's beneficial if you can get to bed before 11pm, as the hot pitta dosha reaches a peak at midnight, so being in bed before this time will help you feel calm and cool, which is always beneficial when you are trying to get to sleep.

2 June

Liven today up with some cross-pattern marching, giving both your circulation and your energy a boost. Start by marching on the spot, bringing your knees up high. If you are steady, as you lift your right knee, raise your right arm up into the air by your ear. Do the same with the left side. Keeping a brisk pace, switch between the sides, stretching up tall. Occasionally, hold the move with your knee and arm up, testing your balance on each side. Now try the same marching move but with the diagonals of the body – right knee high, left arm rises, then left knee high as the right arm rises – again keeping up a brisk pace, holding occasionally.

The cross-pattern movement helps to bring balance to the left and right hemispheres of the brain, so has the added benefit of helping us to feel more relaxed.

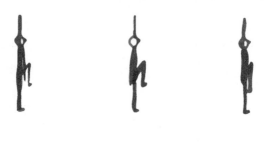

---

3 June

In summer, it's beneficial to focus on food that the Ayurvedic system classes as sweet (e.g. oranges, grapes, butter, rice), bitter (e.g. kale, rhubarb, spinach) and astringent (e.g. apples, broccoli, celery), and food that is light and easy to digest. Make the most of the refreshing summer tastes of lime, cucumber and coconut, whilst starting and ending your meal with some sweet-tasting food.

Ayurveda advises that dark meats such as beef, pork and lamb can be even more difficult than usual to digest in summer, so you might choose to avoid them. Other food that can increase our pitta dosha include pungent flavours (e.g. garlic, onions) and food that is salty (e.g. anchovies, olives, salt) or sour (e.g. cheese, yoghurt, pickles) in flavour.

---

4 June

I firmly believe our hands are channels for healing energy. Sometimes, there's nothing more comforting than a warm embrace, the safety of holding hands or a reassuring hand on the shoulder. We all have healing hands, and we can all channel this energy to help ourselves as well as others.

If you are feeling tired, try resting your right hand on the back of your neck, whilst placing your left hand on your back, in the area of your adrenal glands (mid-back area, bottom end of your ribcage). Hold this for a few slow breaths, letting go of the tiredness and heaviness.

Or, to help alleviate pain, place your left hand on the back of your head and rest your right hand on the site of the pain. Use the exhalation to help you release. Remember, as mentioned on 16 May, where there is pain there will be tightness and tension, so feel the warmth of your hand soothing and relaxing.

---

5 June

I particularly like to do a lying twist to aid my digestive system. Experience has shown me that, if done regularly 20 minutes before eating, it helps to reduce the incidence of indigestion, especially acid reflux.

Lie on your back, on the floor. Bend your knees, with your feet close together. Stretch your arms out at shoulder-height along the floor, with the palms facing down. With an out-breath, allow your knees to relax over the right side, as you turn to look to your left, keeping both your hands on the floor. Inhale, bringing your knees back up. Exhale as your knees relax to the left side and you look to the right. Repeat four times on both sides.

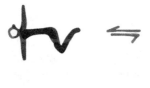

---

6 June

Try this simple posture to help ease the discomfort of heartburn.

Lie on your **left side** with your knees comfortably bent. Use cushions to rest your head and neck on, and your top (right) knee. Rest here for at least five minutes. Lying on your right side has been shown to aggravate heartburn, so here we are working with your body's natural flow and wisdom.

7 June

Mandalas have long been used as a tool to guide us into a meditative state. These circular patterns usually contain geometric designs, which draw the eye, allowing us to focus inwards, leaving the distractions of the external world behind as we dive into the still space within. Not only are mandalas beautiful to look at, but they are also wholly absorbing if you create your own. You can colour these in yourself (you will easily be able to find templates online – there are even mandala colouring books) or you can create your own, which is a mindful practice in itself.

Connect with the beauty of summer by creating your own natural mandala, using whatever you find – shells, flowers, grass, pebbles, twigs, leaves. I find it easiest to start with a stunning centrepiece and work outwards, carefully positioning each element of the design with the reverence that Mother Nature deserves. Not only does this still my mind, but it instils in me a great sense of gratitude and wonder for our earth. I hope you are in a position to "keep" your completed design intact, at least for a couple of days, so you have a chance to look at it again and again, maybe watching it change as nature once more takes control. If it's safe to do so, perhaps light a tealight in the centre of your mandala, providing a focus for some silent sitting and contemplation.

---

8 June

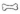

I've already spoken about the restful "child pose" (see 11 February). I'd like to share a couple more variations over the next few days. Today's variation we've met before (see 18 May), but with a little addition that's very useful for taking pressure off your neck or for alleviating a tension headache. I find this variation particularly useful to do before bed, or whenever I need to settle an overactive, anxious mind.

Extended child. Start on all fours. As you lower your bottom towards your heels (you can put a cushion between your bottom and your heels if it's more comfortable), keep your arms extended and your hands where they are. Now try resting your head on a cushion. Rest here for at least five breaths. When you are ready to come out of the pose, walk your hands back towards your head so you can push yourself up.

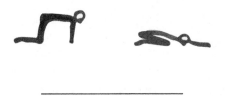

9 June

Taking yesterday's "extended child pose" as a starting point, move into what I have always called, the "banana stretch". This is a beautiful stretch that your back will thank you for, especially if you've been overdoing the gardening!

Start on all fours again. Keep your hands where they are as you lower your bottom towards your right heel, pushing the fingers into the earth to deepen the stretch. Hold for a couple of breaths before returning to the starting position. This will come as no surprise now...lower your bottom to your left heel, again keeping your hands in their original position, pushing into the fingertips for the extra stretch. Return to the starting position and finish with the "extended child pose", lowering to both heels, but this time focus on pushing your fingertips into the earth, giving you a deeper stretch in the broad sheet of muscle that covers your back. I bet you can hear your back oohing and aahing with joy! Feel free to repeat a few more times.

10 June

♡

For a shot of dynamism and a boost to your self-esteem, focus on your manipura chakra at the level of your navel. One of the quickest ways to do this is to practise the sounds associated with this personal power chakra (see 20 May for more information). I like to start with a few rounds vocalising the sound "ah" (as in "rather"). This helps to calm and settle unhelpful negative self-talk. Then, to give you a hit of inner strength and vitality, vocalise the sound "ram", slowly and steadily. You might be able to feel the positive energy of manipura radiating outwards from your navel.

11 June

I have another tip today to improve your balance. This practice strengthens and helps to prevent you going over on your ankles. I like to do this simple exercise whilst waiting for the kettle to boil. Hold onto something, with your feet hip-width apart. Lift onto the balls of your feet, taking your heels off the floor. Hold it steady for a moment, trying not to lift any of the toes, and don't let the ankles collapse inwards, before lowering the heels. Build up the length of time you hold for, and as you gain confidence, lighten the hold you are making with your hands. I find it's easier to do this if I focus on keeping my big toes down, which helps to stabilise my ankles. Repeat until the kettle has boiled!

---

12 June

The classic yoga pose, the "tree", is just the job if you are feeling overwhelmed and unsettled. It helps us feel grounded and centred. As it's a balance posture, it also stops your mind wandering – you need to stay focused on the present moment, otherwise you will wobble!

Start in the "mountain pose" (see 9 January). Pay attention to the connection you make with the earth. With your weight slightly onto your left side, bend your right knee, placing the right foot by the left ankle, with right toes on the floor and your right hip opening out if it feels comfortable (seek advice from your healthcare practitioner if you have a hip replacement). As you inhale, let your wrists float out to the sides and overhead. Your palms are to meet at the top (only raise to shoulder-height, meeting in front of the chest if you have high blood pressure or your shoulders are not happy stretching up). As you exhale, draw the palms straight down the midline of the body to the heart centre. Inhale, turning the fingers to point forwards, still with the palms together, feeling the gentle rise in your sternum. Straighten the elbows as you exhale. Now feel the gentle expansion in your chest as you take your arms out to the sides at shoulder-height, in a wide, embracing movement. Turn the palms to face the earth. Can you feel the polarity with the earth? Bring the hands down to your sides as you breathe out, returning your right foot to the floor. Flow through the arm movements again with the left knee bent. Repeat a couple of times on each side, feeling the connection you make with the earth, rising tall from your firm foundations.

---

13 June

I have a simple yet super-effective tip for alleviating annoying cramp.

Using your middle finger, press the little groove above the top lip, under the nose in the centre. You need to apply a bit of pressure, and sometimes wiggle the finger around until you reach the right spot. Odd I know, but it should ease your cramp almost immediately - trust me!

---

14 June

Today, I write in praise of a piece of dark chocolate. Perhaps not something you were expecting to read in a book about wellness, but nevertheless, dark chocolate is full of antioxidants, which help to protect our cells against free radicals thought to play a part in cancer and heart disease. There's even evidence that dark chocolate can lower blood pressure and improve circulation. Plus, I usually find that a small square of dark chocolate is enough to take the edge off my sweet tooth. Eaten after a meal, it gives us the final sweet taste needed to complete a meal and convince our mind that our appetite is satisfied. Enjoy!

---

15 June

We don't get much moonlight in June, but luckily for us, the full moon of June tends to sit a little lower in the sky so more of its light is able to shine through the atmosphere. This lower position may also be responsible for its pinky red tinge, one of the reasons it is named the "strawberry moon".

Summer, for me, is all about fullness, ripeness and celebrating the beauty of Mother Nature. Although we may not see this moon for quite as long due to the shorter nights, there's more of a chance that the weather might be clement, so you can get out and actually be in the moonlight. If you can get out, take time to connect with the earth. Maybe do some yoga or a meditation – be still. Full moons are a good time to journal. How is your year going? What would you like to see happen for the remainder of the year? It's also a creative time, so a great opportunity to start or complete a creative project. Whatever you do, have fun...and maybe enjoy a moonlight feast of strawberries!

---

16 June

I have another brilliant breathing exercise for you today. "Bhramari" is also referred to as the humming bee breath (the name gives you a clue as to the noise you're going to be making). It is not to be done if you have an ear infection or low blood pressure. Benefits include relieving stress, tension, anxiety, anger and insomnia. It also lowers blood pressure as it is such a relaxing breath, and it supports the healing of body tissue. I've always found it particularly helpful for throat ailments, but best of all, I love it for how it calms my autoimmune responses, so I use it all the way through hay-fever season. Here's a simple version to get you started.

- Sit comfortably. Cover your ears with your hands.
- Inhale through your nose.
- Exhale slowly and controlled whilst making a deep, steady humming sound (like a bee) with the lips still closed and your jaw relaxed.

I like to do five rounds. When I take my hands away, the silence is palpable and my whole body feels nourished.

17 June

If I've been sitting for a while, especially bent over my laptop, I like nothing better than to move into a gentle seated twist, keeping my sternum lifted. If I feel in need of a stronger move, I like to twist from a standing position.

- Place your right foot on the seat of a chair (this needs to be a stable chair), close to the back rest.
- Draw the flesh in away from your abdomen and lift your ribs. As you exhale, turn towards the right.
- As you twist, hold onto the chair with your left hand, allowing your right hand to either rest on your hip or slide around the lower back. On each inhalation, lengthen your spine, and on each exhalation, slowly turn your shoulders to the right, looking over your right shoulder. Allow each out-breath to ease you a little bit deeper into the twist.
- Hold for a few breaths before repeating on the other side.

---

18 June

If I was much younger (and therefore thought myself invincible!) I was given a piece of advice that meant nothing to me then, but means a **lot** to me now. The advice? Look after yourself as if you were 10 years older. Twenty-year-old Isabel did not appreciate the wisdom of this, but a 50+ Isabel most certainly does! I wonder what you make of this wisdom. Today, consider how you would like to feel and look in 10 years' time. What do you want to be doing? What would you like to still be able to do? With each passing year and decade, this becomes more of a challenge. Armed with this information of what you want your future self to be like, find out what you need to do to make it happen!

19 June ♡

The heart – physical, emotional and energetic – is a recurring focus for summer. Self-love, self-worth and compassion for yourself and others are some of the qualities we associate with the heart chakra. We can connect with these qualities and our beautiful heart centre using the "lotus" mudra. Use this to fill your space with love, along with times when you need to love and be compassionate with your Self.

Sitting comfortably, bring your hands into a palm-pressed position just in front of your chest. Keeping the thumbs, the little fingers and the heels of the hands together, open out the middle three fingers to form a cup shape – the lotus blossoming. Simply rest here, breathing naturally, holding the mudra for a few breaths. When you are ready to complete, the lotus gently closes, as you bring the palms back together and thank yourself for the gift you have given yourself.

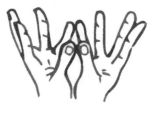

---

20 June ♡

We use phrases such as "digestive fire" and "fire in the belly" regularly. In yoga, though, these are more than just figures of speech, they are relating to the energy of our fire centre, manipura, which gives us the get up and go we need to get things done, and to agni. Agni is our digestive fire, responsible for the digestion and assimilation of all that we eat. There is an adage that goes something along the lines of, "you're as young as your spine and as healthy as your stomach". There is much truth in this. When our agni is healthy, we literally glow with health and vibrancy. When our digestion is out of balance, we feel sluggish, lacking in energy and generally out of sorts. Agni is often likened to the energy of the sun, which is why I mention it here as we reach the longest day. The sun gives us life but, of course, it has the power to destroy. Too much sun is drying, leading to fires. Not enough sunlight and things cannot grow and thrive. Consider today your digestive fire. Think about your appetite, how well you digest food, how you eliminate waste products, and the energy your food gives you. The four types of agni, according to Ayurvedic wisdom, are balanced, irregular, intense and weak. Knowing which one is your prevalent digestive tendency can help you make informed choices about what you eat and how you can keep the digestive fires stoked, without them raging out of control or dampening them down too much.

---

21 June

The summer solstice, the longest day, a day to celebrate summer and the light of the sun. For me, this is a day to practise my yoga and meditation outside. I also like to make sure I get out for a couple of walks, including at the end of the day as the light begins to fade. These jaunts outside give me opportunities to connect with the earth and to give gratitude to the life-giving sun. I'm also fond of a relaxation laid in the sun (living in the north of England, sometimes I need to call on my powers of imagination for this), feeling the warmth of the sun healing and relaxing every cell of my body.

You may well have your own way of celebrating this auspicious day. Perhaps you rise with the sun, acknowledge the sun's zenith at noon, spend time being creative (this is a lovely day to create a mandala - see 7 June - or a sculpture using natural materials), have a celebration summer picnic, honour the light with a homemade suncatcher, or watch it peeping through the leaves of the trees, or play outdoor games in the sunshine. Whatever you do, enjoy it, tune into the exuberant energy of the season, and make the most of the light.

---

22 June

Yesterday, I touched on the healing power of light. There is a beautiful mantra - the "gayatri mantra" - which is all about bringing in light and illumination. You might like to say it at the end of your meditation, or listen to a recording of it whilst in relaxation. Here is the Sanskrit mantra, followed by the translation. The translation is a lovely affirmation on its own, if you prefer not to use the mantra itself.

"Om bhur bhuvah svah
Tat savitur varenyam
Bhargo devasya dheemahi
Dhiyo yo nah prachodayat."

"I meditate on the divine light, the ultimate source of energy that illumines all life. May it remove my ignorance, enlighten my mind, and impart a perfect understanding of reality."

---

23 June

Take some time this morning to just be still.

Give thanks for all that you have. Focus on abundance, rather than lack. Focus on wellness not illness.

Become aware of your heart centre, and feel the gentle rise and fall of your sternum as you breathe. Imagine a light in the centre of your energetic heart (centre of the chest, rather than the physical heart). Allow the light to build in intensity and expand, filling your whole body...healing, relaxing and rejuvenating...filling every cell of your being.

Now let the light shine outwards. Fill your immediate world with light. Can you expand it out into the wider world?

Let's fill our beautiful earth with love and peace.

---

24 June

Last month, I shared with you the classic breathing practice of alternate nostril breathing (see 14 May). This month, I am sharing a variation which is particularly relaxing and great to do if you are struggling to get to sleep. You can do it using the fingers, as I explained previously, or try it when you are laid in bed (on your back will work best), visualising the breath moving between the nostrils. Take a couple of deeper breaths to let your body settle, feeling the breath moving through the nostrils. Imagine or visualise the breath entering the left nostril. Follow its path in through the nostril to the space at the bridge of your nose. Now visualise or imagine the breath leaving the right nostril, following its path again. That's it! Breathe in through your left nostril. Breathe out through your right nostril. Always do it in this direction for this variation. This helps to put you into the right hemisphere of the brain, the relaxation side.

---

25 June   Zzz

Here, I share with you a quartet of simple postures I find effective for sleep, if practised just before I'm ready to turn in for the night. Get yourself ready for bed, then lie down on your back on the floor. Practise each posture for five full deep breaths if you can.

- Start by taking your legs up into the air. You can either let them hang there, all relaxed through your joints, or rest them against a wall or chair.
- Lower your feet, placing them on the floor with your knees bent. On an out-breath, lightly press your spine into the earth, easing out the arch from your lower back. As you breathe in, gently lengthen and arch your spine, so it moves away from the earth. Keep your bottom on the floor as you do this, allowing the arch to extend up to the space between the shoulders if it will. Repeat this subtle spinal wave five times, working with your breath.
- Bring your knees into your chest, holding onto your knees as you focus on pressing your thighs a little more into your torso with each out-breath. You might also like to gently rock from side to side.
- Keeping your knees bent, with feet on the floor and close together, extend your arms along the floor at shoulder-height, with palms down. Allow your knees to relax over to one side as you look to the opposite hand, keeping your shoulders down (you can rest your knees on a cushion if they don't reach the floor). Rest here for five breaths, before returning to the centre, and relaxing over to the other side for five breaths.

When you've finished, you might like to spend a few minutes just lying on the floor, relaxing, focusing on the rise and fall of your tummy as you breathe, before rolling over to sit up, and with as little fuss as possible to your body, getting into bed. Sweet dreams!

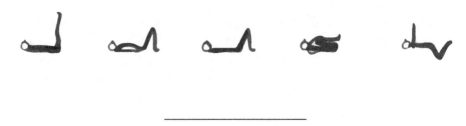

26 June

As we flow through summer, help to keep your pitta dosha in balance with these simple lifestyle changes. Pitta is hot, sharp and penetrating. Coming to the fore in summer, it can raise inflammation and irritation of mind and body. Keep things harmonious by ensuring you have adequate time to relax, avoiding pushing yourself at work or in your personal life. Moderation is key.

- Take cool baths, not sweltering hot ones. Have cooling massages using coconut or almond oil. Avoid sunbathing, saunas and steam rooms. We want to chill out, not sweat it out!
- Rather than one big meal a day, go for four meals a day of smaller portions.
- Choose activities that are non-competitive and relaxing. Shady walks avoiding the midday sun, swimming and cooling yoga are all perfect.
- Make time to relax, be creative and generally do things you enjoy, not things that you feel you must do.

27 June

This is a lovely move for helping us to connect with our heart centre, bringing joy and compassion and enhancing the quality of discernment, something we need in summer when we have so many opportunities open to us. What do we really want to focus on?

Start in the "mountain pose" (see 9 January). Allow your body to be still. Sweep your arms up and over your head into a palm-pressed position (keep your hands at chest level if you have shoulder problems, heart conditions, or high or low blood pressure). Draw the flesh gently away from your pants. Inhale, bending your knees (keep them tracking forwards, not falling in). Exhale, straighten your legs as you bend your arms at the elbows, lowering the hands to the top of the head, still in the palm-pressed position. Inhale, bending the knees, straightening the arms. Repeat, flowing between these moves for at least five breaths. Finish by lowering the arms to your side and being aware of your heart centre.

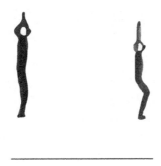

28 June

A wise teacher once advised me to be aware of comparison, which is potentially a destructive habit. It's worth remembering that nobody else is on your path. Nobody else has had your life experiences or sees life from your perspective. Comparing yourself to others is a waste of time, and a waste of energy. What works for one person may not work for another. Try things out, tweak them to suit you and have fun. The key to success is to do whatever you do with sincerity. If something makes your heart sing and makes you feel light-hearted, you are probably on your authentic path, so there is no need to compare yourself with others! If you do find yourself in a cycle of comparison, bring your awareness back to your heart centre, feeling the gentle rise and fall of your sternum. This should bring you back "home".

29 June

Sometimes when I am busy, I take a moment or two out of my day to just be still. I look up at the sky. I focus on the spaciousness and ultimately the infinite beyond the sky. By comparison, everything else seems tiny and insignificant.

Imagine a large and noisy flock of birds. Disturb the birds and they fly away up into the sky, becoming smaller and smaller, until they are tiny dots. Our thoughts are like the birds, gathering and brooding, the noise they make keeping our attention, shielding us from the beautiful blue sky. If we can do something to scatter the thoughts, they will disperse just like the birds, leaving us with the infinite blue beyond. The more we can align ourselves to that which is bigger, changing the perspective of the busy thoughts by shrinking them, the more we can bring in clarity, calm and focus.

---

30 June

When we can concentrate for longer, we bring discipline to our mind, and therefore gain control over what we are thinking. This makes it easier to let go of unwanted, ruminating thoughts. We can improve our powers of concentration with regular practice. Try this simple meditation for strengthening the mind. Sit comfortably in front of an analogue clock, with a second hand. With your gaze relaxed, focus on the second hand moving from 12 round the clock face. How long can you follow it without being distracted by your thoughts? Try just a couple of times in one sitting. We don't want to add any pressure, but do try it regularly, daily, if possible, to make a significant difference. Some days you might struggle to get past a couple of seconds, but as you bring discipline to your mind with regular practice, you will soon notice the length of time increasing. Be gentle with yourself.

You have not failed if the thoughts come straight away. As we've said before, the mind thinks, that's its job! This is a practice to help us find the inner strength we need to avoid becoming consumed by all the thoughts the mind thinks. The mind is a fabulous servant, but a very poor master. Let's remind ourselves that we control the mind, not the other way round.

July

1 July

July, a gloriously vibrant culmination and celebration of all our hard work so far. We are reaching the end of the school year, maybe the opportunity for a holiday, certainly a chance to kick back and relax. A time for frivolity, fun and jolly japes. There is so much going on in summer that it is easy to get lost in the revelry of the season. Keep your energy high by tapping into the wisdom of your heart, cultivating the sometimes-overlooked quality of discernment. Find some balance. Rest as much as you play. Carefully choose which activities you want to take part in. What will bring you the most joy?

2 July

Each new dawn you welcome is a gift. Be aware of this fact – waking up in the morning is a blessing! This morning, take time to enjoy this gift...this present...this present moment. When you first become aware of the new day, enjoy a moment of stillness, giving gratitude for the day ahead and the opportunity it presents. If you get chance, you could take this further. Before the busyness of the day begins, take yourself outside, connect with the earth, touch it with your hands if you can, then look at your hands and imagine you are looking in a mirror, seeing your precious self reflecting back at you. Give yourself a smile. You are glorious and deserving of the best day ahead.

3 July

Wake your body up with these energising moves – they are great first thing in the morning or after you've been sat a while.

Stand with your feet hip-width apart, with your knees soft. Keeping your heels on the floor, start to gently bounce the knees, with the shoulders staying relaxed. Feel the vibrations building and flowing through the body, relaxing your muscles. Now stop. Feel the stillness. Start the bouncing again, still with the heels on the floor, but this time bend one knee and then the other as you bounce. After a couple of minutes, stop. Feel the stillness. Start up again, bouncing both knees together, but this time gently twisting from side to side, as before keeping the heels on the floor. I find this especially relaxing for my shoulders. Now stop. Again, tap into the stillness. By now, you might be feeling your whole body tingling and nicely energised.

---

4 July

Three or four times a year, the planet Mercury goes retrograde, where, for a few weeks, it looks as if it is moving backwards, though in fact this is an optical illusion. It's easy to find the dates of retrograde Mercury, and I suggest you do and take note. Mercury is a planet associated with communication and travel, and often chaos and disruption abound when it is retrograde. If you don't believe me (and it's good to be sceptical), note the retrograde dates and notice if there are any extra travel problems, or maybe upsets involving data or information sharing, or computer issues, and notice the errors in communications and misunderstandings.

With this knowledge we can Mercury-proof ourselves a little bit for a smoother ride.

- Allow extra time for journeys and getting into online meetings.
- Double-check dates and deadlines.
- Watch out for communication glitches, double-checking everything before you send.
- Be careful with your words. If there's a chance your words could be taken the wrong way, you can guarantee that when Mercury is retrograde, they will be!
- Stay clear of harsh words and gossip.
- Speak kindly and develop patience with yourself and others – everyone makes mistakes.

5 July

It's often said that our eyes are the windows to our souls. Wise words. They can also be windows into our general health. I hope you can get a regular eye test. Not only will the optician check your vision, but they will also check your eye health, which can indicate other health conditions. Summer is a good time to focus on our eyes as they can often be sore, itchy and red during allergy season, whilst floaters can be more obvious in bright sunlight. Today, consider your eyes. Show them some love and gratitude. Book an eye test if you haven't seen your optician for a while. If you are a glasses wearer, give them a clean. Take a moment to look at the tip of your nose, and then to a spot in the distance and back to your nose, before allowing your eyes to relax. What do your eyes say about you? Are they the windows you want people to look through?

---

6 July

Continuing from yesterday's optical theme, the eyes are another area of our body where heat can collect (think about how hot and itchy eyes can become when we have an allergic reaction). Here are a couple of soothing things to place over your eyes to bring calm and coolness.

- Slices of cucumber – honestly, this feels lovely, and is great for removing puffiness around the eyes.
- Soak two cotton wool pads in rose water, one for each eye. If it's really warm, you might like to cool these in the fridge before you rest the pads on your eyes.

Find a quiet place to lie down on your back, allowing your breath to lengthen, whilst enjoying the cool sensation and delicious scent of rose water or cucumber, calming the eyes, settling your mind, and softening your facial muscles.

7 July

Here is a move to soothe and relax your lower back. I know it as the "pelvic compass".

Start by lying on your back, resting your pelvis on a cushion so it's a little bit raised. Keep your knees bent, with feet flat to the floor.

Imagine your pelvis is like the face of a compass. Gently rock your pelvis forward and back, north and south.

Now allow your pelvis to rock north-east and south-west, returning to north and south when you are ready. Move now between north-west and south-east, before switching your awareness of the movement to east and west. Finally, finish moving between north and south, each movement becoming more subtle as you steadily come to a still point.

Work through these movements slowly, the rocking movement soothing and relaxing every layer of your being.

---

8 July ♡

Our heart, both physical and energetic, is a recurring theme through our summer wellness tips. Today, let's consider the soothing sounds connected with our heart - the "anahata" chakra. The word "anahata" can be translated as "unstruck sound" referring to the peaceful, harmonious sound that is said to arise from this energy centre when we are deeply connected to universal energy.

Find a few moments to be still. Allow yourself to say out loud the sound "yam". Repeat at least 10 times before being still and silent. Can you feel the gentle vibration in your energetic heart centre? I like to say this sound silently to myself when I feel I need to boost my feelings of self-worth and confidence.

Sometimes, our heart needs calming, perhaps at times of grief when it feels as if our heart is breaking. At these times, try using the sound "eh" (as it sounds when we say "play"), silently or out loud, allowing the sound to soothe and heal.

9 July ♡

In the summer, you might find it beneficial to massage your body after your bath or shower, or before bed with fractionated coconut oil. Coconut oil is recommended to help cool the body. Before bed, pay particular attention to your feet, adding a drop of rose essential oil if this is OK for you to do. It is said to draw the heat down and out, away from your torso, which should help you to sleep. This tip can also bring relief if you are struggling with hot flushes.

---

10 July

Another area to consider massaging, is your abdomen. This is surprisingly soothing, often easing common digestive problems. With a little bit of oil on your fingertips to facilitate the smooth gliding of your fingers on your skin, start by resting your fingers on your navel, pressing gently but firmly. Working in a clockwise direction, keeping that steady pressure, and at a steady pace (don't rush), massage the tummy, each circle you make increasing until you get as high as your ribcage, and as low as your lower pelvic region. Take your time – 30–50 revolutions is great. Now let your hand rest on the solar plexus area (about a hand-width up from your navel). Feel the security that the warmth of your hand provides, before slowly circling this area in an anticlockwise direction. You hardly need to move the hand, keep it resting on the area making a small circular movement. This move brings calm when you are anxious or upset, whilst the clockwise circles work with the natural flow of your digestive organs.

---

11 July

Today, I'd like to share a brace of yoga postures that work perfectly together to support our digestive system, release tightness from the hips and open the front of the torso, helping to take heat out of the body.

- Come into a high kneeling position (rest your knees on some padding). Take your right leg out to the right, with toes pointing forwards and weight rolling towards the little toe edge. Keep your left thigh on the vertical. Don't allow your right leg to stretch too far out – it will nip!
- Let your left-hand rest on the floor (or a block if you don't reach the floor comfortably) by the left knee. Your right arm extends straight up towards the sky (you can keep this arm by your side if it is better for you). This is the "gate pose".

- Now allow your hips to soften, folding as much as you need, so that you can swoop the right arm down towards the left knee then around towards the right, lifting your torso, bringing your right arm to rest along the right leg, the left arm arcing up and over by the left ear if it feels right for you.
- Keep your ribs moving heavenwards, opening the front of the body, in the "beam pose".
- With an out-breath, soften your hips once more, as you lower your left arm towards the earth, letting it come to rest by your left knee, returning to the "gate pose".
- Repeat the flow a few more times, before switching your legs, repeating with the left leg extended out to the left.

If kneeling doesn't work for you, try sitting on the corner of a chair, your left shin on the vertical, foot on the floor, and the right leg extended out to the right. Do the same arm movements as above but resting your hands on your legs or the chair instead of reaching to the earth. You'll still get all the benefits of the postures.

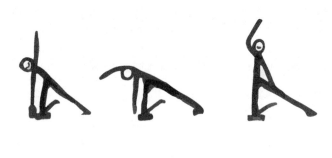

---

12 July

Ayurveda offers guidelines for everyone – not just for our individual constitution – on what, when and how to eat. Some, I find easier to swallow than others (pun most definitely intended!). One recommendation that has always served me well is when to eat fruit. Put simply, the rule is, if you are eating fruit, either eat it alone or leave it alone! Fruit digests quicker than other food, so if it is eaten with other food then it sits in the various parts of our alimentary tract, fermenting whilst it waits for the other bits of your meal to break down. This can cause indigestion and gas. Allow two hours with no food either side of eating fruit. This gives everything sufficient time to move through your digestive system.

13 July

In yoga, we have a couple of fantastic breathing techniques to cool us down, physically and emotionally. Easy to do and surprisingly effective, in my experience they are also handy tools for turning the heat down on a hot flush! (See 14 July too.)

Cooling breath #1 – "Sitali" pranayama

(Not to be done if you have low blood pressure, asthma, bronchitis or excessive mucus.)

Sitting comfortably, allow your tongue to roll into a straw shape. You are either a tongue roller or you're not, it's down to your genes! If you're not, you can just imagine the sides of your tongue rolling up. I'm not a tongue roller so I can tell you it still works. Breathe in through the "straw" you make with your tongue, feeling the coolness of the air as it passes over your tongue into your mouth. Relax your tongue, breathing out through your nose, the heat and irritation leaving the body with the exhaled breath. Work up to nine breaths if it feels OK.

---

14 July

I hope you got chance to practise yesterday's cooling breath. Here's its friend:

Cooling breath #2 – "Sitkari" breath

As with yesterday, this is not for you if you have low blood pressure, asthma, bronchitis or excessive mucus. Also avoid it if you have sensitive teeth, missing teeth or dentures - it might be a bit uncomfortable.

Sitting comfortably, this time gently bring your teeth together, with lips relaxed. Inhale through your teeth, slowly and steadily. Relax your mouth, exhaling through your nose, working up to nine breaths if it's OK for you. As before, have an awareness of the coolness of the breath coming in, expelling the heat with the out-breath.

15 July

The full moon of July is known as the "buck moon", in recognition of the splendid antlers of male deer who will be currently enjoying a growth spurt. The energy of the buck moon is easy and celebratory – a time to relax and kick back – which ties in perfectly with the energy of the month. This is a time to revel in the fullness and creative beauty of the season. Key words to focus on this full moon are **rest, fun** and **joy**. Where and how can you weave these qualities into your July days? Remember to congratulate yourself for all the hard work you've been doing, taking care of your wellbeing this year.

For me, this is also a time to focus on spiritual growth. I like to journal and consider my purpose in life. What am I here to do? I like to check in with the practices I am doing to support my spiritual path. Are they still supporting me? Do I need to tweak my practices or build on something? Do I need to seek further guidance, or perhaps gently pull myself back into line for more consistency in my practices?

---

16 July

Today, I give you the mudra of tolerance. It does exactly what it says on the tin and is a useful little practice when temperatures start to rise! Its classical name is "hakini" mudra, also known as the energisation mudra, but I like this name as it reminds me of the cooperation it brings internally and externally.

Bring your hands together in the palm-pressed position, keeping all the tips of the fingers and thumbs connected. Increase the spaces between the fingers a little, allowing the palms to move away from each other so that your hands are gently domed, forming a pyramid-type shape.

Hold this mudra for at least five breaths (even better if you can hold until you feel your irritation melting away). Best of all, you can do this mudra either quietly on your own, or when you are with people. Notice how many people in the public eye hold this gesture when they are speaking.

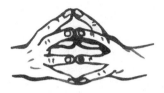

17 July

Crystals and gemstones are not my area of expertise, but I certainly feel their healing energy. One of my favourites is a heart-shaped rose quartz crystal – perfect for the summer/heart connection. Quartz is said to bring balance to all our body systems, whilst rose quartz specifically is reported to transform negative energy, which is probably why I like it by my laptop to soak up all the computer vibes! It is also said to help us find the inner strength needed to deal with unexpected change, whilst enhancing the power of positive affirmations. Who doesn't need a bit of this from time to time? Other qualities attributed to this crystal are its ability to soothe emotional pain, encourage self-forgiveness and acceptance, and promote self-trust and self-worth. If you get chance, have a browse for crystals and gemstones. See, feel and explore their power for yourself.

18 July

Whilst there is potential for us to find stillness anytime, anywhere and any place, sometimes it's useful to consciously make stillness a part of your daily routine. Find a time that works for you and stick to it, even if it's just five minutes lying still in your bed, before you get up. Keep your eyes closed so nobody knows you are awake, if you need to! Have a few moments just for you to be still, to be aware of your breathing, maybe even doing your affirmations. Make this quiet time as much a priority as brushing your teeth or washing – something that you do without question. The more you get into the routine, the more you will benefit and indeed notice the difference when you don't get chance for stillness.

19 July

☆

This is a fun way to test and improve your balance. Walk forwards in a straight line, heel to toe, as if you are walking a tightrope (you can put your arms out like a tightrope walker for extra balance, if it helps). Now try to go backwards. A few steps, go steady. Feeling brave? Can you do it with your eyes closed or partially closed (make sure you're not going to bump into anything)? The trick is to take your time and think about where you are placing your feet. I find I tend to speed up as I get towards the end, but this just knocks me off balance – a lesson for life in general, methinks!

---

20 July

The school summer holidays are just around the corner. A time of year when many of us are heading off to sunny climes or enjoying trips out and about, which can mean a lot of travel time, not many people's favourite part of the holiday. Over the next three days, I have some easy tips to help you travel in comfort, arriving at your destination relaxed and ready to go. Here's the first one:

Keep moving

There's often a lot of sitting and standing around involved in travel, which can make us feel sluggish, as well as not being great for our circulatory system. Counter this by moving whenever you get chance. Move your joints through their natural range. You can even do this when you're sitting.

Flex your toes and feet. Circle your ankles. Swing your lower leg from the knee. Circle around your hips, then try a gentle twist through your spine, and stretch from side to side if you've space. Stretch out your fingers and make fists and release, then circle your wrists. Bend and straighten your arms at the elbows. Gently roll your shoulders forwards, then backwards. Turn your head slowly to one side and then the other. Keep your spine happy with the "seated cat posture". Sitting in a chair, rest your hands on your thighs, round your back by pulling in your tummy and tucking in your chin, then lengthen your spine, moving your ribcage away from your hips, opening the chest and lifting your chin. Repeat a couple of times. Include some hamstring stretches and squats too if you can – great for bringing life back to your buttocks if you've been sat a while!

21 July

Yesterday, I was talking about how to make travelling more comfortable by keeping moving, which is good for our physical health. Today, my travel tip is for our mental health. I don't mind admitting that I am not a happy flyer, but this breath helps to keep my anxiety in check, giving my mind something to do instead of listening to the sounds of the aeroplane.

Calm travel anxiety

First, establish a steady breathing rhythm. If it feels OK to do so, equalise the length of the in-breath and the out-breath. Consciously count the breath in your head. For example, "I am breathing in two, three, four. I am breathing out two, three, four". Gradually start to increase the length of the out-breath, aiming to double it. I still count this in my head. For example, "I am breathing in two, three, four. I am breathing out two, three, four, five, six, seven, eight". You can be as quick as you need to be with the breath, though don't struggle, it should feel relaxed! This will naturally stimulate your relaxation response whilst the counting gives your mind something to think about.

This is useful for any anxiety-inducing situation, it doesn't need to be travel-related.

---

22 July

Yesterday

I don't know about you, but travelling makes me tired, and if you've had to cross time zones, jet lag can be quite debilitating. I think it's worth mentioning that there are plenty of other situations in life that can leave us feeling the same way – shift work, hospital visiting, all-nighters spent with a poorly loved one, or all-nighters spent partying. Here are some things that might help.

- First job, get outside for a walk, or practise some yoga (dynamic if you want to stay awake, soothing and restorative if you want to sleep).
- Whatever time you arrive, it's worth doing a relaxation, even if you feel you should be awake. Lie on your back, on the floor if possible, and let your mind catch up with your body.
- If you want to sleep, do your relaxation in bed, and focus on your tummy rising as you breathe in, falling as you breathe out.

- If you've been travelling for a few hours try out a balance posture (there are plenty of ideas in this book), holding onto something if needed. This helps to alleviate the disconcerting swaying sensation we can feel after travelling, as if we're at sea. Even better if you can do it outside when you're out walking.
- Make sure you are hydrated. Travel is extremely dehydrating.
- I like to place just a spot of the essential oil, vetivert, at the base of my spine. An earthy smelling oil that brings me right back into my feet.

---

23 July ♡

Here is a helpful trio of moves I like to do when my eyes need a rest.

- I start by rubbing my hands together and placing the warm palms over my closed eyes. Then, I draw my fingers lightly together as if I am physically pulling the tiredness from my eyes and flicking it away.
- Then, when my eyes have focused, I look to a point in the distance, before looking at the tip of my nose, repeating this process a couple of times.
- Finally, I look at something soothing yet inspiring, like the flowers in my garden, and let my gaze soften, breathing naturally. Flowers are great for this practice. I honestly feel as if I can breathe in their vibrancy, inspired by their ease. The roses don't force themselves to grow, they just do.

---

24 July

Settle yourself down today for one of my favourite relaxation techniques. This is my go-to practice if I find myself feeling low or I am fed up with myself. I've also used it to great effect at times when I have needed healing (on any level).

Once you are in a comfortable position for your relaxation, you might want to go through a body scan, or a squeeze and release relaxation (see 4 January). Now take your awareness to the soles of your feet and imagine or visualise that you are drawing in the most beautiful, translucent pink light, the colour of a rose quartz. Each time you breathe in, draw this amazing, healing light into your body, taking as much time as you need. Bring the rose pink light into every part of you - your feet, legs, hips, the spine and the muscles of the back, your abdomen and all the organs of the digestive system, into your ribs, chest, heart and lungs, bring it in through your hands, into the arms, shoulders, neck, over the face, the head and to the very tips of your hair – until every cell of your body is filled with this healing, nurturing, pink light. Bathe in the rosy glow and feel your Self being loved.

---

25 July   Zzz

I love all the soft fruits that are abundant in summer, but cherries are my absolute favourite. Not only are they delicious, but they are packed full of nutrients, antioxidants and natural anti-inflammatories, making them a good choice for your joints and heart. They also have a surprising health benefit – they make us sleepy, contributing to a better night's sleep.

Our pineal gland produces the sleep hormone melatonin, needed for its role in controlling our awake-sleep cycle, and cherries are naturally high in melatonin. Try eating a handful (10–20) of cherries for supper and see if it makes a difference to your sleep.

---

26 July   ♡

Take a moment to stand in the "mountain pose" (see 9 January). Bring your hands into a palm-pressed position, in front of your chest. With an inhalation, allow your right arm to stretch up, with the palm towards the ceiling, and the left arm towards the earth, with the palm facing down. As you exhale, bring the hands back to the heart centre, allowing the knees to bend a little. Breathe in, this time moving the left arm up and the right arm down, straightening the legs. Return to a palm-pressed position in front of the chest, bending the knees as you breathe out. Repeat this beautiful heart stretch at least three times on each side. Check you are not forcing the shoulders up – it should be a comfortable, gentle stretch across the chest.

This is a foundation Dru Yoga moving breath, and one of my go-to practices to bring calm and settle an anxious, pounding heart.

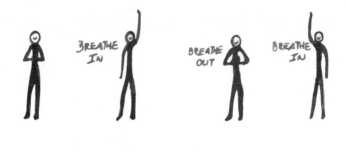

27 July

Roman soldiers were reputed to chew on fennel seeds as they marched, to help decrease any cravings they might have for food. Interestingly, fennel has long been used as an aid for digestion, helping to improve digestive strength. Consider drinking fennel tea or including it in your cooking to alleviate nausea, flatulence, indigestion and constipation. Chew on a few seeds after a large meal to support your digestive system as it works to assimilate the food you've eaten.

It also helps to clear congestion from the lungs (useful if you are a hay-fever sufferer) and is often used in natural toothpastes for its antiseptic properties. Use cooled fennel tea as a mouthwash for sore gums, complementing advice from your dentist or healthcare practitioner.

28 July

Summer is a great time to reach for the stars...or our goals at least! I use Dru Yoga's "archer posture" to help me focus on my target. Take time to consider your goal. Formulate a positive affirmation that encapsulates your dream.

Stand with your feet a little bit wider apart than shoulder-width. Turn your right foot out to the right and let your left foot follow, so your hips are comfortable. Bring your hands to your heart centre, with space between them. Pause here, feeling the gentle rise and fall of your sternum as you breathe. Bring to mind your goal, say your affirmation, visualise it, feel it.

Extend your right arm out to the right, level with your head, with the palm facing away. Bring your left arm up to shoulder-height and, with your elbow bent, form the archer mudra by folding in your ring and little finger, with the middle and index finger extended and thumb pointing up. With an inhalation, pull the left elbow back, keeping the mudra. Bend your back knee, allowing your right arm to rise to around eye level. Again, think about your goal, see it, feel it. With a strong out-breath, let your "arrow" fly to your target by extending the left arm towards the right hand, at the same time allowing your weight to shift forwards, bending the right knee slightly, straightening the back knee, keeping the back heel on the floor. Repeat a couple of times on this side, before repeating to the left. At the end, stand in the "mountain pose", allowing your breath to settle and feel that your positive energy has reached your target.

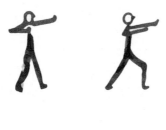

29 July

Connect with your sense of sight by meditating on something inspiring such as a flower. Choose a beautiful flower, one with plenty of petals and a gorgeous colour. Sit comfortably with your flower in front of you at eye level. Allow your breath to settle. Let your eyes relax, settling into their sockets. Allow your gaze to soften as it rests upon your flower. Look at it carefully but without judgement. Be aware of the colour, the shape and the formation of the petals. Observe all the delicate parts that make up the whole flower, and see the subtle variations of colour. Absorb yourself in the beauty of this natural form. Eventually, let your eyes close, spending a few moments in stillness. A flower doesn't force itself to grow, to be more beautiful, it just is, and you can be too.

30 July

The "varuna" mudra is a nifty little move, said to improve hydration to your face and reduce wrinkles.

Connect the top of the little finger with the top of the thumb. Do this with each hand, holding for a few breaths.

That's it! Simple and effective, connecting you with the water element of your body as represented by the little finger. Summer can be quite drying if we are out in the sun a lot, so it's useful to keep the water element balanced. It also helps to soothe cracked lips. You might also want to put it on your winter practice list, as it helps to ease mucous congestion.

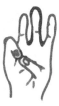

---

31 July

I enjoy this back bend - the "camel" - in summer for the stretch it gives me, particularly appreciating the opening of my chest and the release in the shoulders (perfect if you've been hunched over). Over the years, I have also found it effective in keeping me cool mentally, emotionally and physically.

From sitting — safe for everyone
Sit towards the front edge of a chair. Take your hands behind you, holding onto the seat. Draw the flesh away from your pants, lengthen your spine, with your ribs moving away from your hips. Draw your shoulder blades lightly towards each other, lifting the sternum. If your neck is OK, think about lengthening the back of your neck as you lift your chin, to fully open the front of your body.

From kneeling – avoid if you have spinal problems, digestive problems such as ulcers or a hernia, or a hyperactive thyroid. Kneel on a pad to protect your knees.

From a high kneeling position, as above, draw the flesh away from your pants as you lengthen your spine, with your ribs moving away from your hips. Reach your right hand round to rest on the back of your right thigh. The left hand reaches around to rest on the back of the left thigh. Draw your shoulder blades lightly towards each other, lifting the sternum. See if you can draw the lower part of your ribcage in slightly if it is flaring out. Again, if your neck is OK, lift your chin (don't tip your head back). Assuming no health concerns and you feel comfortable and dynamic, go further by tucking your toes under and work towards resting your hands on the backs of your heels (or use blocks either side of your feet to rest your hands on). Keep your tummy muscles engaged, your inner thighs working (imagine you are zipping them up) and your tailbone directed towards the floor, not sticking out behind you or tucking under you. This is a strong move, so please only do it if you feel 100% comfortable and secure.

To come out of the kneeling position, firm your bottom, lifting the hands. Now lower to your heels and fold forwards into the "child pose" (see 11 February) and rest here for a couple of breaths.

August

1 August

I flow through August with an awareness that there is no more work to be done. Mother Nature has reached her verdant and ripe pinnacle, and for this year at least, the growing season is over. I say this not to be downcast but rather with great gratitude for all the abundance present in my life. As late summer approaches, I think this is the perfect opportunity to reflect on how your year is progressing so far. Be grateful for the gifts, the lessons, the opportunities that have come to you (sought or unsought). Check you are still heading in the direction you want to go in, and your thoughts and actions are still in harmony. Take time to reassess, realigning if necessary.

2 August

I hope you love this joyful breath as much as I do. Even saying its name fills me with joy. "Surya pushpam" – the sunflower breath. A breath to calm and uplift.

Lie on your back with your knees bent, with feet together. Interlace your fingers and let them rest into your lap with the palms facing the thighs. Inhale, taking the arms up and overhead, keeping the palms facing away from you and the fingers interlaced. Exhale as you bring the arms back to rest in the lap. Coordinate breath with movement.

Once you get into the rhythm, add in leg movements. As you inhale, the arms move up and over, and at the same time let the knees fall out to the sides, bringing the soles of the feet together. On the exhalation, bring the knees back up as well as the arms back into your lap. The arms and legs are to reach their destination as you complete the breath, so the arms will need to move quicker than the legs, which is a great practice for cultivating calm and body awareness. Don't rush though, as you settle into a few more rounds.

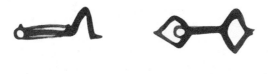

3 August

We have many states of being, connected with the heart – we can have hard hearts, lion hearts, heavy hearts, cold or warm hearts. Today though, let's consider the quality of light-heartedness – a quality I often think is overlooked, but I find is essential for my emotional wellbeing. It's so easy to be weighed down by the troubles of the world that we forget to enjoy ourselves. A smile can say so much, an attitude of cheerfulness can change the energy of a room and the people within it, and I like to think the potential to change the energy of the world around us. More than anything, though, I urge you to laugh at yourself! There really is no need to take ourselves so seriously. Nothing destroys the ego more effectively than having a good old chuckle at our idiosyncrasies.

4 August

I've only recently discovered the joys and benefits of a rebounder (mini trampoline), but I'm hooked now! I find that five minutes bouncing boosts my circulation, encourages my shoulders to relax, plus I've discovered it is helping to tone my waist area! It also makes me smile, which is reason enough to practise in my opinion.

Start with some gentle bouncing, with heels down, knees soft and shoulders relaxed. This might be enough for you. If you feel dynamic, try some bouncing with the heels off the floor, then perhaps lifting the feet into a little jump. Maybe add in some twisting or scissor the legs and arms (forwards and backwards, then in and out), or perhaps a bit of jogging on the spot. Play around with the moves and have fun.

When you are ready to finish, take your time to slow down, before coming to a standstill. Hold onto something to steady yourself as you step off your rebounder – you can feel a little bit wobbly if you're not used to it.

---

5 August

As early in the day as you can, take a moment to just be, to stand on the earth. If you can do this outside then even better, maybe barefoot so you can feel the grass or the sand beneath your feet. Bring your hands into a palm-pressed position with the thumbs on the sternum. Be still and welcome the day with gratitude.

- Moving at your own pace, allow your arms to extend forwards, opening the palms up. Imagine the sun rising, right there on your palms.
- Soften your knees and inhale, taking the arms up and overhead slowly. When your arms reach the top, let them separate, opening wide, with palms facing the sky. Tilt your face up to the sun, allowing yourself to bathe in the light.
- Now with an out-breath, softly fold into a forward bend, bringing the hands just about level with the knees, easing the back into this move.
- As the backs of the hands come together, bend your knees, pushing into your feet as you uncurl into standing, taking the arms up the midline of the body then up and over as in the second bullet point.
- Relax into a forward bend again, perhaps taking the hands as low as the shins. Uncurl as before.
- Relaxing forwards again, maybe this time you can let your hands touch the earth. Pause here. Feel the length from tailbone to crown. Let your legs lengthen. Connect with the cool, stillness of the earth.
- When you are ready, bend your knees again, uncurling into standing for the last time. Stretch up, completing by bringing the hands back into the palm-pressed position, with thumbs on the sternum.
- Once more, return to stillness, the only thing moving is the gentle rise and fall of the breath. Feel that you are perfectly positioned between the heavens and the earth. Affirm your connection with the earth, rising tall from your firm foundations, reaching for the highest.

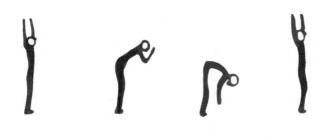

6 August

When the temperature is rising, there's nothing more appealing than an ice-cold drink…but wait a minute! A warm cup of tea might be more refreshing. Our body has a core temperature (around 37°c), which it likes to maintain. If we drink something very cold this can give our internal systems a bit of a shock, forcing the body to work harder to get the temperature back up to what it is comfortable with, so we could actually be making ourselves warmer. A warm (not too hot) drink though, will stimulate our body's cooling response, such as sweating, so could well be a more cooling option in the long run. Try it and see how you feel.

7 August

Yesterday, I mentioned you might want to try a warm drink during the summer months to keep you cool, refreshed and hydrated. Why not give some of these herb teas with cooling properties a go? Choose from peppermint, liquorice, fennel or rose. They taste as delicious as they smell, plus they are caffeine-free, so great for helping you to relax. You can also rest the cooled teabags over your closed eyes for an instant refreshing eye bath – I love a two-for-one deal!

8 August

We have a beautiful practice in yoga where we withdraw the senses, called "pratyahara". This helps us to conserve and harness our energy as we are not wasting it on the vagaries of the senses, whilst bringing us back to our centre. It's also a great lead into a relaxation or meditation. Spend a little time today noticing your senses and perhaps where they lead you. No judgement or criticism, just bring gentle awareness.

Can you focus on each of the senses? Touch, hearing, smell, taste, sight. Is one easier to connect with than the others? Or indeed trickier? Be aware of how the senses distract us. I only need to hear a song on the radio and it takes me right back in time, away from the present moment. If I catch the smell of fresh roasted coffee, I can hear cake calling me and then I have a real battle on my hands to bring me back to the present moment – and it's the present moment where I might make a more conscious decision as to whether I really do want a sweet treat. This is how the senses can grab us, leading us into aversion and attachment, and the whole mind melodramas that go with, and before we know it, we've frittered away some of our vital energy. Are you aware of any specific sense memories that take you away from the present moment?

9 August

Yesterday, I talked about the practice of pratyahara (sense withdrawal). Today, I invite you to try a relaxation (lying down) or a meditation (sitting up) using this technique.

Find yourself in a comfortable position, taking a few deeper breaths to let yourself settle. Become aware of the connection that you are making with the earth – all the places of your physical body that are in contact with the earth. Move your awareness now to all the places of your physical body that are in contact with clothing, being aware of the different weights, textures and pressures, and all the places not in contact with clothing. How does the atmosphere feel against your skin?

Now become aware of the sense of hearing, searching out sounds outside the room you are in. Then become aware of the sounds within the room and finally bring your awareness to the sounds your own body is making.

Leaving the sense of hearing, become aware of the sense of smell. Without judgement, how does the atmosphere smell? Move your awareness to the sense of taste. Can you taste the last thing you ate or drank, or maybe taste the atmosphere on your lips?

Finally, become aware of the flow of your breath. Watch it as it enters your nose and nostrils, into the body and the lungs. Where does the in-breath become the out-breath? Watch its path out of the lungs, the body, the nose and the nostrils into the atmosphere. Where does the out-breath become the in-breath? Be a curious observer, the seer of the breath, not trying to alter it, just allowing each breath to take you a little bit deeper into stillness.

---

10 August

You can strengthen the arches of your feet, strengthen your toe joints and even help ease the discomfort of plantar fasciitis, with this simple sitting position. Perhaps surprisingly, you'll also find it beneficial for your digestive system.

Start by sitting in a low kneeling position so that you are sat on your heels (rest your knees on a cushion if it is more comfortable), with your toes tucked under. See if you can stay sitting on your heels for a couple of breaths, thinking about lengthening your tailbone (so you are not sticking your bottom out or tucking it under) and being aware of the breath moving in the abdomen. This might feel a bit tricky at first as your toe joints are probably not used to being in this position, so build up slowly. Come out of the pose if it is painful.

Now try rocking back, lifting the knees, keeping your hands on the floor for support and the bottom low to the heels, then lower your knees to the earth again. Repeat a few times. This is great for maintaining the movement in your toe joints.

---

11 August

According to yogic wisdom, lying on the right-hand side is more relaxing than lying on the left. When you roll onto your right side you effectively close the right nostril, allowing you to breathe more fully through the left nostril. This, in turn, activates the right side of your brain (your relaxation side), potentially leading to the slowing down of the heart rate and a natural lowering of blood pressure. This further ties in with the practice of alternate nostril breathing that I shared earlier (see 14 May and 24 June). If you are struggling to switch off at bedtime, try relaxing on your right side first.

---

12 August ♡

Today, I am sharing a most beautiful mudra that emulates the shape of the lotus flower, a stunning flower that rises from the murky, muddy depths of the pond, just as we rise from the depths of our sometimes murky emotions to fulfil our potential. Use this mudra to connect with your heart centre, the wisdom of your heart, and the power of self-love and approval.

Sitting comfortably, bring the backs of your hands together. Allow the little fingers to link, then the middle fingers and the index fingers, leaving your ring fingers and thumbs free, so that you can connect them lightly on each hand (i.e. the tip of the right ring finger touches the tip of the right thumb, and the tip of the left ring finger touches the tip of the left thumb) forming a two-petal lotus flower. Hold the mudra in front of your heart centre for at least five breaths, breathing slowly and deeply, before releasing.

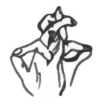

---

13 August

The heat of summer can aggravate our fiery pitta dosha, which has a detrimental effect on our digestive system - it's one of the reasons many of us suffer with upset stomachs when we are on sunny holidays. To keep my digestive system moving steadily and my digestive organs cool, I like to practise a simple sitting side-stretch.

Sit on your bottom, with your legs outstretched as wide as feels comfortable. You can sit on a cushion if it is more comfortable. Can you keep your knees and your toes pointing up towards the ceiling in this starting position, firming up your inner thighs? Allow yourself to flow, gently stretch from one side to the other, your following hip rolling a little so that the movement always feels nice for your back. As you stretch to the right, let your right hand slide along the leg, then the left hand eases down the left leg as you ease towards the left side. Make sure you don't push further with your hands, this should feel relaxed, bringing movement into the side of the body. After a few rounds, you might want to hold the stretch. Slide towards the right, with the right arm relaxed, and if it feels right for you, let your left arm stretch up and over towards the right. Gently spin your ribcage towards the ceiling, so you focus on a side-stretch rather than a forward bend, and keep your shoulders relaxed. Soften and relax into the stretch for a few breaths before repeating on the other side.

Finish by bringing your legs together, bending the knees and giving them a hug.

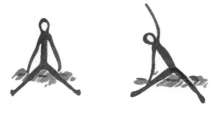

---

14 August

I love this playful move. It soothes my nerves and relaxes my spine. I practise it before bed to help me sleep, or when I come in from a busy day and need a quick rejuvenation. It also helps me to tap into the inner-child energy that can so often get lost in the busyness of the adult world.

- Lie on the floor, on your right side (make sure you have plenty of space to roll into). Arms out at shoulder-height along the floor. Knees bent.

- Breathe in, sweeping your left arm up and over. Feel that you are opening your chest area as the left arm comes to rest at the left side. Try to keep your knees together, still on the right side.
- Now lift the left knee, moving it away from the right leg, steadily – don't rush. You will get to a point where you begin to roll onto your back and the right leg starts to lift. Try to keep this distance between the knees. As you roll over to the left, the left knee gently lands on the floor at the left side. Allow the right knee to join its friend so that only your right arm is left on the right side.
- Once both knees are over, then finally we draw the right arm up and over until it rests on the left arm.
- Now roll back onto your right side, in the same relaxed, yet mindful way, each limb moving separately. This is one complete round. Repeat as many times as you wish. I usually find three is enough to change my energy.

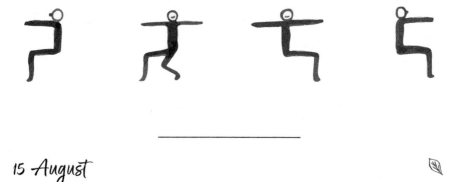

15 August

The full moon of August is named after the prehistoric looking fish, the sturgeon, which abounds in the Great Lakes of the US at this time of year. As we've already seen, summer is a time for showing off, flourishing, enjoying the fruits of our labours. As we approach the end of the season, our thoughts might turn to themes of harvesting and reaping, having gratitude for all that we have. Take some time this full moon to consider the following, maybe meditating or journalling to help you get the information you seek.

- Remember all the things and people you are grateful for. If you have the chance, say thank you to the people who bring you love and joy, who have helped and supported you through the year. If you don't see these special

people in person, then maybe write them a thank you note – I assure you it
will be joyfully received.

- Is there still a goal or dream you would like to fulfil before the autumn
leaves fall? What action can you take today to move that forward?
- Autumn is a fabulous time for letting go of what no longer serves us (more
on this later), so now is the time to consider areas of your life where you are
not following your heart. These are maybe areas where you might be open to
change, perhaps you are ready to let go of habits, thought patterns or even
people that no longer align with your values.
- The full moon is always a good time to connect with water (the moon
affects the water balance of our body, just as it affects the water tables of
the earth). If you have spent time considering the point above, it may have
brought about anxiety. As you connect with the water (either physically
or through visualisation), imagine your anxieties and fears being washed
away, carried far away by the flow of the water – let them go.

---

16 August

Summer is a beautiful time to connect with nature – it's easier to be outside at this
time of year than on a cold, wet winter's day. Connecting with nature brings calm,
and a sense of perspective. One of the joys of summer, for me personally, is that it
brings the opportunity for some quiet time, sitting outside.

Sometimes, I hold a pebble (or a shell) whilst I sit in my silent reverie. As I connect
with the feel of the stone, I find that life is gently put into perspective. I am just like
the pebble, a very small part of a huge picture. My time on earth is minimal, unlike
the mountains that have been here for millennia. My problems are like the small
pebbles, not important in the grand scheme of things.

If I'm lucky and by the sea, I watch the waves. Each individual wave breaks free, then
peaks and returns to its source, always part of the ocean. I may think I am separate
but one day I will return to the earth.

Other times I lie on the ground, watching the passing clouds. How beautiful to be
able to flow and change with the ease of the clouds, and I am reassured that the
blue sky is always there, even if the clouds cover it for a short time.

On a clear night I look at the stars. A visual reminder of my own mortality and of the spark of the divine that I believe we all are, and I am soothed.

---

17 August

Release the tight grip of a tension headache with a couple of simple self-massage moves. Start by lightly resting your fingertips in the centre of your forehead, and with gentle pressure, slide the fingers out towards the temples. Return the fingers to the centre of the forehead but a couple of finger-widths higher, again sliding them steadily with even pressure out to the sides. Continue to repeat the sliding motion with the fingertips, moving a little bit higher each time, as you work backwards over the scalp. Finish by softly tugging small tufts of your hair, working all over your scalp. Take a few breaths to be still and have a drink of water, before returning to your day.

---

18 August

This simple yet effective exercise will help bring awareness of your deep core postural muscles. Lie on your back on the floor, with your knees bent and your feet flat to the floor. Draw your pelvic floor up towards your spine and gently draw the flesh of the lower abdomen away from your pants. You might feel your lower back flattening to the floor. Try not to force this and keep your natural spinal curve, if you can. Hold for 10 seconds, breathing naturally. Release and relax. Repeat 10 times, every day if you can. Remember, the aim of this exercise is not to tire yourself out as if bracing yourself for impact, but to bring gentle awareness and engagement to these muscles.

19 August

Building on yesterday's exercise for bringing awareness to our core postural muscles, today we can move a bit further, by lifting and lowering each vertebra from the base up, one at a time, with strength and control. Lie on your back on the floor, with your knees bent and your feet flat to the floor, arms to your sides on the floor, with your palms facing down (you can use your hands for support if you need to).

As you breath in, press your feet into the earth, engaging your lower abdominal muscles (as we did yesterday), lifting your bottom from the floor, lowering as you breathe out. Inhale, lift the bottom and the next vertebra up, lowering as you exhale. Continue in this way, working up the spine, right up to the shoulders if you can. How many of your vertebrae can you feel lifting and lowering independently? When you've finished, let your legs stretch out or hug them into your chest and rock – listen to your body to see what you need to do.

This is our "bridge posture". The perfect pose for improving the health and flexibility of your spine. It's also a good summer practice, as it helps us to connect with our heart centre.

Stay with yesterday's posture. If you have rheumatoid arthritis or neck problems, or an overactive thyroid gland, check with your healthcare practitioner before practising.

---

20 August

I have another variation of yesterday's "bridge posture" (as before, with health considerations). Again, this will benefit your back, helping to build the muscles around your bottom that support your pelvic girdle.

Start in the "bridge posture", lifting all the way up to the top if your back and neck are OK with this, keeping your neck relaxed. Once your hips are raised high, make sure your buttock muscles are working as you roll the weight to the outer edge of your feet, so that your knees relax out to each side. Now draw the knees back in, placing the feet flat to the floor again. Repeat 10 times if you can, keeping your hips high as you move, so that your gluteal muscles are working.

---

21 August

Last month, we used sound to bring balance to the heart chakra, anahata (see 8 July). The heart has been a continuing theme throughout summer, so let's delve a little deeper into the beautiful heart chakra. Resting in the very centre of the chest (we don't focus on the physical heart), this chakra is all about being open to love, joy and compassion, for ourselves, for others and for our world.

- Be honest, on a scale of 1–10, how much do you appreciate yourself and others? If you are scoring low, what can you do to improve this? My advice is start by listing all the things you are grateful for, then move onto listing the qualities and achievements you love about yourself and admire in others.
- Make a point of saying something kind and/or positive to everyone you meet, and at least once a day to yourself! For example, "I like your jumper", "Thank you for your help", "How can I help you?", "I really enjoyed your interesting presentation", "What is that lovely perfume you wear?". People remember how you made them feel long after you have gone.
- Emerald greens will help to bring balance to the heart chakra, whilst pinks will soothe and calm. Wear, surround yourself or get creative with these colours.
- Use a rose quartz crystal to bring balance to anahata.
- Love yourself by using delicious floral-scented essential oils in your bath, in your moisturisers or in oil burners. If they are OK for you to use, choose from rose, ylang-ylang, jasmine or neroli.
- Take a moment to be still. Feel the gentle rise and fall of your sternum as you breathe, allowing a sense of spaciousness to develop. Dive into the stillness.

22 August

Sometimes, we all need a little soothing. When my nerves are feeling jangled, I turn to this relaxing breath, the breathing equivalent of being given a reassuring hug. You can do this lying, sitting or standing, just find yourself a little time to be still so that you can focus on your breathing. Let your breath settle and deepen, and when you feel ready, try the following ratio. Inhale for a count of seven (go as quick as you need to with the count). Rest and pause the breath for a count of one. Exhale for a count of seven (same pace of counting as the inhalation). Pause for a count of one. Continue with this ratio for as long as you feel comfortable, working up to 10 rounds if you can. Remember, the pauses are just that – you are not holding the breath, just allowing a natural rest before the next part of the breath. Feel the gentle rise and fall of your sternum as you breathe. Be aware of a natural expansion at your heart centre.

---

23 August

When the pitta is rising, it's easy to become irritated and hot-tempered. As someone with a sharp tongue, this tip, given to me by one of my teachers, has been invaluable!

If in a potentially volatile situation, before you speak take a mouthful of cold water. Hold it in your mouth until it warms up to body temperature, before swallowing.

This takes the heat out of your words, whilst giving you enough time to think about what you are saying. My wise dad would often say to me, "Isabel, engage your brain before you engage your mouth". I understand now what he was getting at and, more importantly, how I can do it.

---

24 August

If you are good at standing on one leg, make it a bit more challenging by standing on a folded blanket. Do hold onto something if you need to though, you can always start to relax your hold as you steady. This will help to improve your balancing ability, plus the muscles you use for balance will have to work a bit harder for you to remain stable on this more unstable surface, bringing strength, particularly, into your feet and ankles.

25 August

Your ears might not be top of your "areas to massage" list (what do you mean you don't have such a list?!), but why not give them a little treat today with this stress-busting mini massage? It's surprisingly relaxing, plus it can alleviate headaches, ease muscle tension and give your energy a boost.

First remove earrings, then using your index finger and thumb, gently squeeze and release all the way around the rim of your ear, giving the lobes a little extra squeeze and tug. Move back up to the top of your ear, applying light pressure around the grooves below the ear rim, tenderly pressing into and releasing the areas of cartilage. Now press your finger into the flap where your ear connects to your head, as if shutting out the noise, then release. Finally, take hold of your ears, gently pulling outwards, so that you feel a slight stretching sensation in the area behind the ears, then pause for a breath before releasing. Before moving on with your day, take a couple of minutes to be still and enjoy the warm glow of your ears.

---

26 August

Earlier in the month, I talked about resting on your right side to help you relax. Good advice - I hope you tried it!

In yoga, we also recommend lying on your right side if you overheat in bed. If we're having a good summer, this may well be useful to know. You might have noticed this yourself. I naturally prefer to sleep on my left-hand side, but if it's a warm night, I always find myself rolling onto my right. In yoga philosophy, the left side of the body (open when we lie on the right side - see 11 August) is the cool moon side.

There is also such a thing as getting out of bed the wrong side. Keep that feeling of calm by rolling onto your right side first when you come out of your relaxation time. If you really need to wake yourself up though, maybe if you find it difficult to get up in a morning, try rolling over onto your left side, opening the more active sun side of your brain.

27 August

Sometimes, we need help to rise above the melodrama of life and react to each situation from the truth of the present moment, rather than from the conditioning of the mind.

I love standing in the "mountain pose" (see 9 January), using the Dru Yoga "gesture of humility". Extend the index finger of both hands, folding the other fingers in with the thumb. Bending your elbows, bring your left index finger to the right shoulder, and then the right index finger to the left shoulder. Rest here, affirming to yourself, "I have all the inner strength and resources I need to navigate the play of life smoothly and easily". It can be no other way!

Use this mudra to give you the clarity to focus on what is important.

---

28 August

One of the things I have always loved about yoga is the awareness it brings to every part of my body, encouraging me to take a holistic approach to my health and wellbeing, to take time to listen to my body, discovering what it needs. One thing I soon became aware of – inspired by the teachings of Vanda Scaravelli in her influential book, *Awakening the Spine* – was the bias I had for the front of my body, seldom paying any heed to the back of my body.

Try this awareness from either standing or lying on the floor on your back (or, why not try both and see if there are any differences?!).

Take your attention to the back of your ankles, let the heels sink into the earth, creating space in the area of the Achilles tendons. Connect with the earth, become grounded and settled. Let your awareness rise from your firm foundation, settling now on the back of the knees. Let them extend. The knees spend so much time in a flexed position, they will welcome this opportunity to release.

Move your awareness to the hip girdle. Create space at the back of the hips, noticing the stability this brings. Feel that you are supported. This, in turn, brings a lightness through your spine, allowing the area at the back of the waist to lengthen.

Consciously take your breath to the back of the lungs. If you are laid on the floor, can you feel your back moving against the earth as you breathe? I particularly enjoy this move and the ease it brings to my breathing.

As the back of the neck lengthens, feel a gentle pull along the back, your skull perfectly placed atop the spine. From here, feel the area at the back of your skull relax. I find this a most exquisite and indeed unusual release, but extremely relaxing. Let your eyes close so that you can't be distracted. Give your eyes permission to relax back into their sockets.

How was this exploration of the back of your body? Did it reveal anything? Remember to give thanks to the back of your body.

---

29 August

Are you hungry? Are you *really* hungry? I, like many others, am a comfort-eater, but deep down I know that I rarely feel better for indulging, after the initial rush of pleasure, because I always go for the sweet treats! I now try to be more mindful of my hunger and ask myself a few questions.

First, I check to see if I am thirsty. It's the same sensation. Sometimes, a cuppa is all I need. If I find myself still wanting food, I ask myself if I really am hungry. Is my tummy grumbling? When did I last eat and did I eat enough good quality food? Or is there another reason? Boredom, emotional upset, stress, hormonal? I can tick all these boxes at some point. I find it's good to be aware of where my mind and body are at. If I suspect I am desiring food not because I am hungry but because of an emotional response, I try to be still for a few moments. I take a few breaths deep into my abdomen and ask what the hunger is telling me. It's worth getting used to the sensations. True hunger is a growl that comes from a very different place to emotional or boredom hunger. The more you practise, the easier it becomes to notice the difference and make a discerning choice. If you are not hungry, take time to ask what your body needs instead of food – is it support from a friend, yoga, a walk, some relaxation or creative time? This is all great fact-finding for our personal wellness map.

---

30 August

When was the last time you said something kind to yourself? I honestly believe that every cell in your body listens and responds to the messages you are giving it. During a period of intense ill health with an autoimmune condition, I came to recognise the power of self-talk, for good or bad! I discovered that I had lost faith in myself, I didn't trust my body and I was cross with myself for being ill, repeatedly punishing myself with the harsh words I used about my body, my illness and what my mind was telling me was failure. It was quite a journey to discover that what I actually needed to do was to love myself more, to speak kindly to myself and show my body that it was worth listening to.

This is a huge subject, with many books written about it. I encourage you to explore them, to see if any of them resonate. Most of all though, I encourage you to speak kindly to yourself. I've given ideas for positive affirmations throughout this book – give them a go! Maybe start with, "Dear body, I am sorry for the pain I have caused you with my intentional and unintentional toxic words. I now speak kindly and lovingly to you, and I thank you for the way you always support me and give me life".

If you don't believe positive self-talk will work for you then why not try it and prove me wrong? At least you'll know then! What have you to lose?

---

31 August

Sound, vibration and music have been used for millennia to lift our mood, to help us relax, to soothe the soul, to heal and to connect with spirit. Research has shown that music and vibration have the potential to benefit our health, with modern science proving what the ancients always knew, that sound is frequency, and we are just the same.

You probably already know what sort of music you like. Why do you like it? How does it affect your mood? Maybe try some different genres of music, see how they affect you. Make yourself a playlist of your favourite uplifting tunes and your most relaxing sounds.

Explore the healing sounds of different ancient philosophies, such as chanting, drumming, singing bowls or gongs. There are plenty of recordings on the internet, or maybe you're lucky enough to experience a live sound bath. Immerse yourself in the nurturing and healing vibrations of these traditional musical delights.

September

1 September

September – a month that heralds autumn as we return to school and work after our summer break. It can be a busy time, but see if you can find moments throughout the month to notice the subtle changes in the energy, the weather and in the natural world as we edge into this transitional season.

Transitional seasons generally offer us opportunities to take stock, let go and reassess our health and wellbeing. Now is the time to consider if you need to make any changes to your routine to ensure you have the reserves you need to stay healthy through winter. You might want to make notes on this in your journal. Be open to some of the autumn Ayurvedic lifestyle and diet suggestions I'll be making over the next few months, preparing for the stillness of winter, once it arrives.

2 September

It's easy to convince ourselves that we don't have time to sit quietly or do a relaxation. We don't need lots of time though. Even short bursts of stillness, or a conscious awareness of letting go, are beneficial. In my experience, it's the continuity rather than quantity that is key. Sometimes, we just need to be imaginative about finding still time – waiting for a friend, standing in a queue, waiting for the kettle to boil, being still in bed for a few moments longer before you open your eyes.

Today, see if you can find yourself a couple of minutes to be quiet and still. Get into the habit of finding yourself these rejuvenating pockets of spaciousness throughout your day. I promise, it will be worth the effort.

3 September

Autumn can upset the balance of our "vata" dosha, so this month I will be sharing a few easy things we can do to restore balance. I like to start by understanding the energy of the season and discovering what signs I am looking for that might indicate imbalance.

The vata dosha is dry, windy and airy, which we can certainly see reflected in the season around us.

Some common signs to look out for showing that vata is running a bit high are heightened anxiety, dry skin, problems with static (you know, when you get a shock from the supermarket trolley!), bloating, constipation, IBS symptoms, cracking joints that might feel a bit stiffer than usual, feeling lightheaded, insomnia. If you are nodding your head at any of these, then rest assured, I've tips coming up in the next three months to help.

---

4 September

Autumn is the perfect time to give a little more thought to how you breathe – even better if you can spend time practising some of the yoga breathing techniques I've been sharing, many of them focused on bringing calm, clarity and steady energy to our day. Start and finish your day with one of the following, depending on how you feel:

- To bring calm and soothe jangled nerves – deep yogic breath (see 31 March).
- To bring balance to mind, body and emotions – alternate nostril breathing (see 14 May).
- To help you breathe more easily – "pigeon breath" (see 30 March).

---

5 September

According to Ayurvedic philosophy, we need to tweak our diet again for autumn, favouring food that is sweet (e.g. wheat, rice, sweet fruits, squash, butter), sour (e.g. pickled vegetables, vinegar, lemons and limes) and salty (e.g. olives, anchovies, sea vegetables and sea salt). Focus on meals that are nourishing, warming and easy to digest – now is the time for comfort food!

Avoid cold and/or raw food and drink, ice in drinks, and beans, all of which can aggravate the vata dosha and disrupt our digestive system. It's worth noting, whilst a little bit of fermented food is beneficial for digestion, too much can provide heat and might lead to indigestion or irritation in the body, as well as increasing the production of mucus.

---

6 September

Cross-pattern movements help to naturally ease us into our relaxation response, so try a couple of these moves after a busy day to help you reset:

- March on the spot, bringing one knee to the opposite hand, switching between sides. You can bring your elbows to your knee if you're feeling dynamic. Try to bring your knee across the midline of your body to get the full cross-pattern effect – it also helps to support your digestive system.
- Now take your feet behind you (one at a time) to touch your hand to the opposite ankle.
- How about doing one knee and one ankle (i.e. right knee to left hand, right hand to left ankle)? Once you've got it, switch sides!

---

7 September

As we slowly make our way towards winter, September is a time when I start to think about giving my immune system some extra support, and I usually start with a favourite affirmation. I can't take the credit for coming up with the words, but it has been in my repertoire for so long, I must apologise for not being able to remember its origin.

"Every cell in my body vibrates with energy and health. I nourish my mind, body and soul. My body heals quickly and easily."

---

8 September

You can help to develop strength and stability in your torso with this variation of the "cat posture". The extension of the arm and leg will also work on your balance.

- Start on all fours, with shoulders in line with wrists and hips in line with knees. Rest your knees on a blanket for comfort.
- As you breathe in, stretch your right arm forward as you lift it up to shoulder-height, turning the palm to face inwards, reaching out with your fingers.
- At the same time, lift your left leg, extending it behind you, so your straight leg is parallel to the floor, with your toes pointing to the floor and your heel pushing away.
- Hold this position for about five breaths. As you lengthen your spine, including the back of the neck so your crown is extending forwards and the tailbone is lengthening backwards, still reaching through the limbs, keep your pelvis in a neutral position and your navel gently drawn in towards your spine, giving your torso stability. This is a beautiful stretch!
- Release and repeat with the left arm and right leg. Repeat five times on each diagonal.

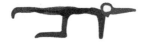

9 September

Anyone else's knees feeling stiff and creaky? My knees very much enjoy a bit of TLC during the colder months with this soothing massage that stimulates the production of synovial fluid to lubricate the joints, whilst relaxing the surrounding muscles.

Sit with your legs extended. Imagine your right kneecap is a square. Place your thumbs at the top corners and fingers at the bottom corners, lightly moving your kneecap forwards and backwards a few times, before resting your thumbs across the top of your kneecap (on the thigh, not on the actual kneecap) and your fingers running along the sides of the kneecap, gently rolling the fingers from side to side for a subtle sideways movement of the kneecap.

Using your thumbs, make small gentle circles on the muscles around the knee joint, not on the kneecap itself. Massage the thigh muscles, round the side of the knee and on the area of the shin, working lightly as these areas can be tender. Now use your fingers to massage the muscle at the back of the knee.

Finish by clasping your hands at the back of your thigh, to support the leg as you stretch it out, then bend the knee a couple of times, before switching legs.

---

10 September

Here's a great movement to help remove fear.

- From standing, rest your hands on your back around the kidney area (between the lower ribcage and navel). Even better if you can make fists and hold them in the kidney area.
- Keeping your hands in this position, start to bounce up and down on your heels, keeping your toes on the floor and your knees soft and not locked out.
- Bounce at least 20 times. If your legs start to feel like lead, give them a shake out.
- Affirm to yourself "Within me is all the courage and inner strength I need".

Bouncing on your heels has the added bonus of helping to keep bones dense.

11 September

Apart from the foods I mentioned earlier in the month (see 5 September), here are a few more food stuffs that aggravate our vata dosha and are good to be aware of, as we move into autumn. If you overindulge on these foods, you might find your emotional state becomes more anxious, or you find yourself a bit more creaky than usual. They can also leave us bloated as they increase the wind element within our body.

- Yeast
- Refined sugar
- Tea, coffee and caffeine drinks
- Very spicy food.

It's also worth noting that two of the biggest culprits for draining our immune system are stress (which can be aggravated by caffeine) and sugar. Being mindful of what we eat pays many dividends.

---

12 September

Sitting just below the diaphragm and a little to the right of centre, at the top of your abdomen, rests your liver, a vital organ responsible for many essential functions, including the removal of harmful toxins and waste products from your digestive system. The hardworking liver is amazing, very forgiving of the pressure we put it under, and even capable of a certain amount of regeneration. The liver is also a big heat producer, so it will come as no surprise that when the liver overheats, we can get a bit irritable or snappy (hence the term "liverish" to describe a crotchety person). Following the heat of summer, moving into the flux of autumn, your liver might appreciate extra support. Here are a few ideas worth trying if you are feeling irritated (physically, emotionally or mentally) or your digestive system is not running as smoothly as you would like.

- Be mindful of what you are consuming. Eat food that is easy to digest, avoiding heavily processed food and drink. You may choose to avoid alcohol.
- Check whether the liver-supporting milk thistle is suitable for you to take. I notice the benefit of taking this mostly in my digestive system.

- Imagine bathing the area of your liver in the most beautiful emerald/leafy green, to soothe and calm.
- Try making the sound "cha" if you find anger or jealousy are rising – both emotions are linked with the liver.

------

13 September

Autumn is a time when joints can start to stiffen and crack, so it is a perfect time to take your joints through their natural range of movement, to encourage the production of synovial fluid to lubricate them.

Sit on the floor, with your legs extended (sit on something if you need to). From here, work systematically, moving your joints through their natural range, doing each exercise four times if you can. Here is a quick run through.

- Toes – curl and stretch them out.
- Ankles – flex and extend, and then rotate one way then the other.
- Knees – hold at the back of the thigh, bend the knee, and straighten the leg out, trying to keep the foot off the floor.
- Hips – bend the knee, with foot on the floor so that you can open out to the side and back up. Now take hold of the foot and support the knee with the other hand. Move the hip by bringing the leg across your body and out. Once you've done these moves on both sides, bend both knees and, with feet together, allow your knees to move out and down and then back up.
- Fingers – make fists, then extend the fingers.
- Wrists – flex and extend. Now make fists and rotate them one way then the other.
- Elbows – arms out in front at shoulder-height, flex and extend. Do the same with the arms out to the side at shoulder-height.
- Shoulders – hands on shoulders, rotate the shoulders one way then the other.
- Neck – turn your head slowly to each side, then allow your ear to move towards the same shoulder on each side. Finish with your chin moving slightly forwards and down, then uncurling the neck, gently raising the chin, so that you have described a circle with your chin.

Don't mind the creaking and cracking, it's just the air being pushed out of the joint cavity, the pressure rebalancing. Clunking is not so good though – stop if you hear this and get it checked out.

---

14 September

Overeating can be problematic for our digestive system, not to mention our waistline. In the west, perhaps we have lost our way somewhat when it comes to portion size. One way to measure your portion size is to cup your hands together – this is about the size of your stomach. In yoga, this is called an "anjali". Ideally, our breakfast would fit into one anjali, with another anjali for our evening meal, with the biggest meal of the day at lunchtime filling two anjalis. This way we are not overloading our digestive system.

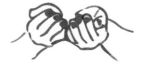

---

15 September

It perhaps comes as no surprise that the full "harvest moon" of September is focused on giving thanks for all that we have, and letting go of what no longer serves us. It's very much linked to the autumn equinox and the agricultural harvesting that traditionally happens around this time.

As always, the full moon is the perfect time to turn inwards, to find some stillness to reflect and to meditate. Start by giving thanks for all that you have – in particular, things connected with your home. Abundance is a recurring theme of September, so consciously seek it out, especially in the natural world. Maybe you will be inspired with a creative project. You could make a natural mandala (see 7 June) using autumn treasures – conkers, acorns, berries and leaves. Then spend some time considering what you are ready to let go of this season. I like to physically write these down, as it helps me to focus, and as I do so I give thanks for all that these things have given me (the lessons, the labour-saving help, the joy etc.), before I ceremoniously rip up the paper. If it's a cool autumn day, I then throw it on the fire, symbolic of the letting go process – I'm all for a dramatic gesture!

---

16 September

Autumn offers us the opportunity to settle into a new rhythm. A slowing down, preparing for the stillness of winter and the chance to let go – the natural energy of the season. We can learn a lot from the trees as we flow through autumn. Watch how they put on the most resplendent display of colour, a fabulous joyful celebration, showing gratitude for the leaves that have served them so well during spring and summer. Then, without fuss, regret or attachment, they simply release them to the earth. Autumn is the perfect time for us to celebrate, show gratitude and lovingly let go of habits, thought patterns, belongings and anything else we no longer need. Be open to this possibility and what it might mean to you.

---

17 September

It's not always easy to say what we really want or need to. Expressing ourselves effectively is so important for good mental, emotional and physical health. Focusing on the throat chakra, "vishuddhi", could well help you communicate more easily. Working with the throat centre is also great if you are wanting to express yourself creatively.

- Strengthen your voice with some singing.
- Take time to listen to your inner voice – you need some quiet time to hear and learn to trust your intuition.
- Observe yourself when you have conversations with others. How much are you talking? How much are you listening? Practise listening – really listening – not thinking about your next words.
- Wear a palette of turquoise, aqua, light blues and misty blues, the colours of the throat chakra.
- If you like gemstones, turquoise is the gem to work with to bring balance.
- If it's OK for you to do, add a drop of relaxing lavender essential oil to your bathwater or body cream.
- Give the humming bee breath a go (see 16 June).

18 September

Although it's easier to relax lying on your back, due to the connection of the sacrum area and the back of the head and neck with the earth, which stimulates our relaxation response, relaxation doesn't have to be done lying down. Get into the habit of checking in with your body at regular intervals throughout the day. Scan from the toes to the top of your head, notice how each part feels, notice where you are holding onto any tension. You can then use the squeeze and release technique, or imagine light coming into the area of tension, consciously asking your body to relax as you breathe out. Or maybe just close your eyes for a few moments and visualise yourself in your favourite place, somewhere you can rejuvenate and be at peace – how does it feel, sound, smell? – coming back from your micro holiday when you are ready.

---

19 September

Autumn is all about change, which is not always easy and can bring up all sorts of emotions, thought patterns and habits, not all of them helpful. Sometimes, it feels easier to stay as we are. This is when it's important to have a clear idea of why you want to change. It also helps you to keep moving forwards, be consistent and make small, incremental changes. Here are some ideas to help you keep going when things get tough.

- Start your day with a positive intention. Let this intention guide your day.
- Be clear on why you want to make the changes. What is motivating you?
- Do something for the good of someone else, every day. Notice how it makes you feel.
- Practise your skills of self-discipline. Consider a habit you would like to break and commit to not giving into it for a week – it's just seven days. Alternatively, commit to not doing it for one day a week for seven weeks. Be gentle with yourself though. If you lapse, no problem! Forgive yourself and try again. I promise you'll get a lot further if you are kind to yourself.
- Practise gratitude. For anything and everything, including the habit you want to let go (it served a purpose once upon a time) and for your inner strength helping you to move forwards. In my experience, gratitude awareness is never wasted.

20 September

Yesterday, I briefly mentioned gratitude. Indeed, you might have noticed it pop up a few times throughout the year. Cultivate this powerful, life-affirming quality with a gratitude journal. Start your day off in one of the most beautiful ways by jotting down a few things you are grateful for...whatever makes you smile or brings comfort (e.g. waking up this morning, good health, a warm cup of tea, the sun shining, being able to read and write). Alternatively, end your day on a positive note with things from your day that fill you with gratitude (e.g. the person who left a space for you in the traffic queue, your feet that have carried you around all day, your comfy bed, a relaxing bath). Gratitude lists are lovely to read through when you're feeling fed up – they remind us that there's always something to be grateful for.

---

21 September

Today is the International Day of Peace. Peace must start with us. We may not be able to influence world events or even things happening closer to home or within our family, but we have complete autonomy over **our** thoughts, words and deeds. By taking responsibility and focusing on peace within us, finding the peace that always rests within our hearts, we send out ripples of peace – to our family, into our community and out into the world.

Here are a couple of my favourite things to do to nourish the peace within:

- Every morning I light a candle for peace. This not only sets the tone for the day, reminding me of what is important, but it also gives me a focus for meditation or quiet time.
- Meditation. Sitting quietly, allowing my mind to become peaceful, so I can focus on my heart.
- In challenging situations, I visualise everyone and everything involved being surrounded by love hearts (I am a very visual person). If there is disharmony, every time I think negatively of the person or situation, I imagine doves flying to them carrying words of peace. I know this sounds a bit way out, but honestly it works! Try it and prove me wrong.

22 September

The big hip joints can get quite stiff if we don't keep them moving comfortably through their full and natural range. Tight hips can be painful and limit mobility, as well as cause problems in the knees and the back, so it is good to keep them lubricated with movement, if you can. From a holistic viewpoint, the hips can represent our ability to move forwards into our future. Hips often get tighter and less mobile as we get older. I wonder if this is because we get more afraid about what life has in store for us? Why not try these seated moves for starters? If you can sit cross-legged on the floor, do so (notice which leg is to the front), if not sit on a chair or sit on the floor with your legs outstretched so you are comfortable and stable. Feel free to sit on a cushion.

- Start by making small circles with your hips in one direction. Slowly and steadily, increasing the size of the circles if it feels OK. Do the same number in the opposite direction.
- Take one arm up by your ear, allowing yourself an easy side-stretch over to the other side. Can you feel the space between your hips and ribs extending on the top side, and a gentle squeeze on the side you are moving to? Ease back, before repeating a couple more times on this side. Now do the side-stretching to the other side.
- Allow yourself to fold forwards. If you are on a chair, you can rest your hands on your thighs as you relax forwards. If you are sat on the floor, you might find you are not moving very far forwards, which is perfect. The idea is to soften into the forward fold, allowing your hips to relax downwards, so absolutely no pushing or forcing!
- If you are sitting cross-legged, do the above movements but with the other leg in front now – you may well notice a difference between the sides.

---

23 September

Nothing keeps me awake more than worrying about not sleeping and how tired I will be in the morning! I have spent many a night clock-watching, waking up in the early hours, anxiously watching the minutes and hours tick away. Then I learnt about natural sleep rhythms, which have honestly revolutionised the way I think about sleep.

We sleep in 90-minute cycles, naturally waking after this time. Sometimes, this is just the point we change position and go back to sleep, or we need to use the bathroom and hopefully drop back off again when we return to bed...but other times this is when our mind can sneak in with all those niggles and concerns, and before you know it, you are tossing and turning unable to settle. Prior to the industrial revolution, we were much more in tune with our sleep patterns, going to bed when it was dark, rising at dawn, accepting those wakeful times in the night. This is when people would get up and maybe read, have a drink, tend to the fire, make love or have peaceful conversations. The industrial revolution, however, brought the need for sleep to be more regulated to fit in with the shift system way of working, and I suspect, brought with it worry about not sleeping! Next time you wake up maybe try getting up, make a drink, read something relaxing, write your ruminating thoughts down in your journal (often, just writing them down takes them out of your mind) and break the cycle of lying awake with the mind churning thoughts over and over.

---

24 September

Have you felt the turn of the season? You might sense that the earth and the elements are rapidly changing as we move through this transitional season. Just as we did in spring (see 27 March), find some time to be outside and connect with the elements. Affirm your connection with the earth, feel yourself grounded and stable, totally supported. This can be especially useful if you are feeling anxious. Draw strength from the earth. Seek out any connection with water in the atmosphere or in your body. This can be a little trickier in the dry autumn. Do you need to drink a bit more, eat seasonal produce or maybe indulge in a nourishing oil rich massage? Can you still feel the warmth of the sun? Maybe think about taking vitamin D if there is not much sun about - a useful support for your immune system as we move into winter. The element of the wind is probably more tangible at this time of year. You might have noticed your joints creaking a bit more, your skin drying, your digestive system being more erratic, possibly with bloating or constipation.

Be still and connect with the season. Ask your body what it needs to be in harmony with the season, to bring balance to the elements as they flow within and through you. Take time to witness and enjoy this beautiful, colourful season, which seems to change daily.

25 September

Back thinking about hips again today! Hips can get tight when we are sitting for a long time, so give them a pleasing stretch with a "seated warrior".

Sit on the corner of your chair, turn so that your right knee is in front, bent at 90 degrees, and your left leg extends behind you, giving a wonderful stretch in the front of your left hip. Feel the tone in the legs, draw the flesh away from your pants and lengthen your tailbone. Place your hands on your front thigh and take a few breaths as you allow your shoulders to relax. If you want a deeper stretch, lift the left arm up by your ear, continue to breathe deeply, lengthen your tailbone, move your ribs away from your hips and open your chest. Repeat on the other side.

---

26 September

Heart symbol

I am a big fan of a cold shower. This is a practice gaining in popularity, with evidence showing how it supports our immune system by giving us a bit of a shock, thus spurring the body into action. A cold shower helps to clear stagnant energy from my aura, making me feel "alive". You don't need to stay under for the whole of your shower – just a quick blast of cold water is enough either at the end or the beginning. Personally, I like to do it at the beginning. I step into the shower whilst the water is still warming – this way, I know the warmth is coming! If you are new to the way of the cold shower, my suggestion is to ease yourself in, initiating your limbs for the first few times, then bits of your torso, gradually building yourself up to a full immersion (you may never feel you want to fully immerse yourself).

Avoid sudden exposure to cold water if you have heart problems (existing or at risk of developing).

27 September

Today I offer a simple lying twist to aid the digestive system, useful for when digestion isn't flowing as smoothly as it might and you are feeling bloated. It's also effective at easing reflux if you do it 20 minutes before you eat. Also practise it if you've been sat for a while and your lower back has stiffened up.

Lie on the floor on your back, with your legs extended. Bend your right knee, placing your right foot on your left knee. Allow your right arm to extend along the floor at shoulder-height to anchor your position. Take a light hold of your right knee with your left hand (no problem if you only reach the thigh). Keeping your right shoulder connected with the earth, gently draw your right knee over to the left. It might not get very far, which is fine. Keep your right shoulder in contact with the floor and do not tolerate any pain. Pause here, using your out-breath to relax a little further into the twist, feeling the stretch in your right buttock. Ease back up to the centre, stretch the right leg out, and when you are ready, repeat with the left foot on the right knee, holding the left knee with the right hand.

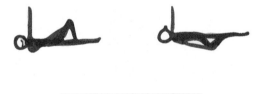

---

28 September

Have you ever tried the technique of introspection? Done regularly, this can be an effective tool for change. I find it helps me let go of any ruminating thoughts that always seem to appear at bedtime.

- Before you go to sleep, spend a few moments either sitting or lying down (if you can stay awake) to reflect.
- Quickly review your day, hour by hour. This is just a scan through, so don't get caught up in emotions or events.
- If you notice an interaction that was negative, change it to a positive. How would you have liked this interaction to have played out, so it benefited all involved?

- Repeat each evening, for at least a week, and see if you have made simple changes to how you react.

---

29 September   Zzz

I always know when my vata dosha is out of balance because insomnia rears its ugly head. I also know I need plenty of sleep to keep me well, so I've learnt many techniques over the years to help me get a good night's sleep.

One of the most useful tools in my insomnia toolkit is the "shakti" mudra. Fold your thumbs into the palms, holding them in position with the index and middle fingers. Outstretch the ring and the little fingers. Bring the hands together to touch, allowing the tips of the ring fingers and the tips of the little fingers to touch. I hold this mudra before I get into bed, holding for about 10 breaths. I also find it useful to do if I wake up in the middle of the night and can't get back off to sleep.

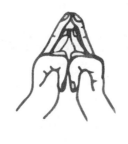

---

30 September

I have a gloriously playful and relaxing move for you to try today – the "happy baby"!

Start by lying on your back. Bring your knees into your chest and rock gently from side to side, before extending your legs up into the air, with knees relaxed. Take your arms up in to the air too, with shoulders relaxing down towards the earth and elbows soft. Dangle here for a few breaths. You might want to stay like this, but if you feel like moving, have a play around – circle your wrists and ankles in both directions, stretch your legs up, sway a little from side to side. Try these last two moves whilst holding your feet. However you feel like moving, keep it relaxed and enjoyable, and feel your body soften a little with each move.

October

1 October

We are well into autumn now. It's easy and understandable to feel melancholy as the light fades and, of course, in October we turn the clocks back. This year can be different though! Look for the silver linings as the nights draw in, our signal surely to move into a new rhythm of life. Let us settle into and welcome a slower pace. We can take our time making nourishing meals – join the slow food revolution. Sleep and rest a little more. My favourite thing about the longer evenings is that it gives me time to explore indoor creative pursuits. Maybe you have a hobby you've been wanting to take up, a jigsaw to complete, or perhaps you have some reading or study to catch up with. Nurture is your watch word for October, so whatever you do, make sure it delights and brings comfort.

2 October

The Dalai Lama was once asked to sum up in one word what the secret to happiness was. I wonder if you can guess his answer?

It was **routine**.

This may surprise you, but if you think about animals, babies and young children, routine is very important to them. They are happiest when their essential needs are met at regular times. The spaces in between the routine bits can then be filled with fun.

Routine is also highly regarded in the Ayurvedic tradition, and never more so than in autumn as it helps to calm the wind/air elements, restoring harmony.

What do you think about routine? Could you see it helping you? Where could you build routine into your lifestyle? Remember, the point here is to meet your essential needs as efficiently as possible, so you can have more fun.

---

3 October

If these darker nights are making you feel a bit miserable, cheer yourself up today with some "gorilla walking". It is also effective at warming you up.

With your feet a good shoulder-width apart (adjust as necessary), fold forwards, taking hold of your feet with your hands, so that you're stood on your fingers and your thumbs are over the tops of your feet (if you can't reach your feet, hold your legs in a way that works for you). You can only move now by lifting your feet with your hands! Do a few stomps on the spot to get into it, now walk forwards, then back. How about to each side? Play around, have fun. I challenge you to do this without smiling!

---

4 October

I've mentioned in earlier tips how autumn can disturb our vata dosha, so today I am sharing a few ideas how we can keep ourselves in balance. Vata likes routine and regularity, whilst disruptions to schedules, eating at odd hours and irregular sleeping habits can all cause imbalances, so focus on:

- Eating at regular times
- Not skipping meals
- Getting up and going to bed at the same time each day
- Keeping to a steady, manageable work schedule – take regular breaks and factor in time for fun, leisure and exercise
- Keeping warm.

5 October

Here's a simple tip for helping you to feel calm and present – **smile**!

The brain cannot tell the difference between a spontaneous smile and an intentional one, so whichever you are doing it stimulates the same pleasurable, relaxed feelings. A big smile that involves the muscles around your eyes and not just the corners of your mouth (you know, a grin from ear to ear) has been shown to lower your heart rate significantly following a stressful event, being effective even if you are not feeling happy. It's the muscle activation that's important. Try it now...go on! Bring the corners of your mouth towards your ears...right up, that's it. Let the smile extend into your eyes. I hope it's made you feel brighter. Remember to smile at the next person you see, even if it's you in the mirror – I bet you get a smile back.

---

6 October

What we eat and drink can significantly affect our anxiety levels. First thing to think about is cutting out or at least reducing caffeine (perhaps you can replace with herbal teas, hot water or warm milk) and sugar. Make sure you stay hydrated, as dehydration will cause you to feel anxious, because the body will think it's in danger. Eat a varied diet of fresh food so you get the B vitamins, magnesium and calcium, and essential fatty acids. It's worth remembering too that alcohol – though it may seem like a relaxing friend – in the long term can increase anxiety.

---

7 October

The "ganesh" mudra can be of special help when we need to find the inner strength to let go, focus on what is real and move forwards with courage. Ganesh is the elephant-headed Hindu god of beginnings, said to be the "remover of obstacles", with the strength and courage of an elephant to clear the paths for us.

Hold your hands in front of your chest/heart area, with your left hand nearest to you, with palm facing away and thumb down. With your right palm facing you, hook the fingers of the hands together, with elbows pointing out towards the sides. As you exhale, keeping the fingers locked together, gently pull the elbows out to the sides, feeling a slight engagement of your chest and upper arm muscles.

You can close your eyes if you feel safe to do so, holding the mudra for a couple of minutes. You might like to make a positive affirmation too such as, "I flow easily with life" or "I deserve the very best".

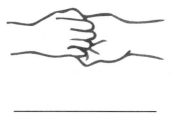

8 October

I have to be honest, today's tip might take a little bit of getting into, but perhaps you'll think it worth a try! Warm about 50ml of sesame oil (assuming no allergies) and hold it in your mouth, swishing it around the teeth and gums for a couple of minutes before spitting it out – make sure you don't swallow the oil! This practice, known as oil pulling, is said to help keep the mouth healthy, being particularly beneficial for the gums, supporting good dental hygiene.

9 October

It's not always easy to make the right choices for our mind and body, as other things get in the way of our good intentions. Keep affirming to yourself, "I make the best decisions to uphold the health of my mind and body". I use this to stop me making impulsive decisions. It gives me the time I need to make a mindful, rather than a mindless, decision.

10 October

Try this variation of the "cat posture" to ease a stiff back. I also find it to be particularly useful when my nerves feel a bit sensitive. Make sure you work mindfully, as you don't want to cause any irritation.

Start in the classic cat position on all fours, flowing through a few rounds (see 19 February). Hold the position with your tailbone tucked under for a breath or two, before allowing your chin to extend gently forward and rise, keeping the rest of your spine rounded. Ease back if it feels uncomfortable.

Lengthen your spine, again, pausing here, with your awareness on the engagement of your lower back and lower abdomen, supporting your spine, making sure you don't dip your lower back too much. Gently relax your head and neck so your chin moves in towards your chest. Hold this for a few breaths if it feels comfortable.

Finish with a few flows of the original "cat posture" to relax, maybe lowering your bottom to your heels to give your back a stretch.

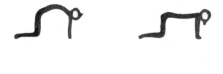

11 October

For me, autumn is a season that makes it easy to cultivate an awareness of the natural cycle of life. Spring is all about new shoots, summer is about growth, in autumn we harvest, whilst that which is no longer needed dies off, and in winter, Mother Nature rests, preparing for the cycle to start again with the light and optimism of spring. Embrace this cycle as it is an essential part of life. Celebrate the season. Give gratitude for all that you have (take inspiration from harvest festivals), have an autumn clean, get out your woolly jumpers, cosy up with blankets and warming drinks. Make your home a place you'll be happy to hibernate in. Autumn is the season for nesting!

12 October

Way back on 28 February we practised a useful exercise for keeping our digestive system moving smoothly. Sometimes, we need a bit more help to ease the passage of waste products through the large intestines, particularly in autumn when constipation can set in. This is when a variation of the aforementioned posture can be useful.

As before, start by lying on your back, with your legs outstretched if you can. Bring your right knee into your chest, as you **exhale**, holding round the shin with both hands. **Inhale** as you raise your head from the floor (this is causing more abdominal pressure, which quite literally pushes the waste products along the large intestines). Lower your head on your next **exhalation**, finishing off the flow by stretching the leg along the floor as you **inhale**. Repeat four times on the right side, then four times on the left side.

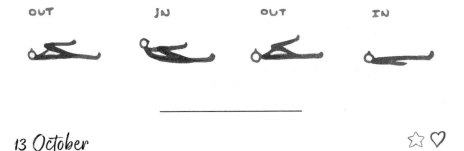

13 October

Today, I invite you to cultivate the quality of curiosity – it keeps you young! Learn something new every day. A new word, a phrase in a different language, the name of a wildflower, a new recipe, a new dance...the opportunities are endless. Even when you are tired, still make yourself learn something. Have you noticed how worlds shrink as people get older? Keep pushing out, keep your world expanding, and the muscles of your mind flexed.

14 October

Warming food and drink is the order of the day in autumn. Try this vata-soothing "elixir" when you feel in need of nurturing or grounding.

On a low heat, bring to the boil the following:

- One cup of milk of your choice.
- A quarter of a teaspoon of turmeric.
- A quarter of a teaspoon of ginger powder.
- A small pinch of cinnamon, cardamom and black pepper (if you are struggling with sleep, you might want to add a little nutmeg too).

---

15 October

October's full moon, often referred to as the "hunter's moon", offers us another opportunity to let go of what no longer serves us as we head towards the end of the year. This is the perfect time to start a meditation practice, so find yourself a quiet corner, warm and cosy. Have your journal handy for any insights that might appear after your quiet time. Focus on your breath until you settle, then contemplate:

- What has this year taught you so far?
- Is there anything you would have liked to have done differently?
- What would you like to let go of?

This is a safe, private space for you to be honest with yourself, without judgement.

Maybe you would like to find pictures or images that appeal to you. Stick them in your journal. What messages are these giving you? Do you need to do some research and look for information that will help you move forwards? Today is a good day to do these tasks.

---

16 October

It stands to reason that our throat area, in holistic terms, is all about our ability to communicate and our power of self-expression. If you are having trouble making yourself heard, speaking your truth, or you feel unable to express yourself creatively, try working with the sound "ham". Say it out loud, say it quietly, say it silently, letting the vibrations of the sound resonate throughout your being.

If you tend to talk too much, overshare, or express yourself in a pushy dogmatic way, you might find it soothing to work with the sound "ee" (as in the word "free"), which can bring calm to a very busy area of our body.

---

17 October

Taking your arms overhead, interlacing your fingers and lifting your ribcage can help to ease the discomfort of constipation. Make this an even more effective move by kneeling on the floor, with your toes tucked under, then sitting back on your heels – a move we first came across in summer (see 10 August). It's not the most comfortable, I must confess. However, you might want to try it, as not only does it help your digestive system but it also helps to strengthen your toe joints. You can put some padding between your bottom and your heels if it's more comfortable.

Raise your arms up and overhead, interlacing the fingers, stretching up. Lengthen your tailbone, lifting your ribcage away from your hips so you are creating space at the back of the waist – plenty of room for your digestive organs. You might be able to feel the movement of your diaphragm as you breathe, massaging your large intestines, aiding the passage of food through the gut.

---

18 October

Maybe you've noticed your mind has a habit of being noisy the minute you sit down for some quiet time or meditation. I find it helpful to organise my thoughts by journalling, which helps to still my busy mind. We looked at journalling at the start of the year, so flick back to 6 January if you need a reminder. There has been much written on the whys and wherefores of journalling, but all that matters is that it works for you. One thing I would suggest, though, is that you ask yourself questions such as:

- Why do I behave like this?
- Why is it that I am really good at x?
- What is it I need?
- Which is the right path for me to take?

When we ask questions, we may not have the answers straight away, but if you put your thoughts, questions and contemplations down on paper, you may well find the answers present themselves either during the silence of meditation or the next time you are journalling. Wisdom comes from many places, and not always in the order you would like it to be presented. Don't worry about this now. All you need to do is be open to it and write down whatever occurs to you. Imagine a jigsaw puzzle, and the picture is you. Each nugget of wisdom you receive is like a piece of the puzzle you can place. There might be a piece missing for quite some time, but trust that it will come.

---

19 October

Settle yourself down for a different type of relaxation today. As always, make yourself comfortable, ensuring you are warm enough, and perhaps going through the physical squeeze and release of muscles, systematically relaxing through the body (see 4 January). Once you feel your body still, bring your awareness to the natural flow of your breath, feel it lengthen and deepen as you relax a little bit further with each out-breath. Make a gentle humming sound as you breathe out – it's not loud or forced, more of a subtle expression of contentment, like a cat purring! Let the ripples of vibration expand, flowing into every cell of your body. Now consciously direct the vibration to any areas that are still feeling tense – where there is resistance or tightness, or where there is pain. Feel the area releasing, dissolving the pain or tension with each out-breath. Spend the last few minutes of your relaxation in stillness and bathe in the silence.

Gentle vibration can be deeply relaxing and healing. Try this relaxation technique and experience it for yourself.

20 October

It's around this time of year that the clocks go back in the UK. I love this and relish the extra hour all to myself. For me, it's all about the extra hour in bed, which fits with the energy of the season, plus I still have plenty of time to do what I want.

What will you do with your extra hour? Whatever you decide, please spend it doing something for you, something that brings you joy, that nurtures mind, body and soul. Allow yourself to flow naturally through the day, don't resist this change of the seasons. Where there is tension or jarring, there will be resistance and stagnation. Be open to the dance through the seasons and literally "go with the flow", bringing grace and ease to your days.

---

21 October

As we move through autumn, heading towards winter, go with your body's natural desire for more sleep. Rising with the sun is always a good cue, whilst the energy of the earth is still calm and peaceful. At the other end of the day, get to bed as early as you can, to give you plenty of rejuvenation time and help you fight off seasonal bugs. During the day, try to get as much light as you can to keep your circadian rhythms (internal body clock) in harmony. Check out the tips for sleep throughout the book if you have problems.

---

22 October

We can use our breath very effectively to ease a path through resistance. Resistance may show up as physical pain, but it could just as easily be emotional resistance, or a persistent unhelpful habit.

During quiet time, observe the resistance. Where do you feel it in your body? Breathe into this area and imagine it expanding with the breath. Pause and feel the resistance. If you are working with pain, see if you can time the pause to the pinnacle of the pain if it is going in waves. Now breathe out, releasing the tension, the resistance, the pain. Just as we don't need to hold onto the old, stagnant breath, we don't need to hold onto these old stagnant thought patterns, emotions, habits, whatever it is causing the resistance.

Focus on the breath, expand and let go. This is a breathing exercise to return to time and time again.

---

23 October

I love this coordinated breath and movement flow to help me feel grounded and centred – the perfect antidote to jangled nerves. It's also a great sequence for easing stiff joints.

Start by standing in the "mountain pose" (see 9 January). Bring your hands by your navel, with palms uppermost. As you breathe in, draw your palms up towards your throat. As you breathe out, turn your palms down and straighten your elbows so you can push them towards the earth. On your next in-breath, turn your palms to face outwards, raising your arms up and overhead, letting the hands separate at the top. As you breathe out, let the arms float down to your sides and back in front of your abdomen so you can flow through the sequence again.

Keep this flow going, coordinating breath and movement. Feel an expansion as you inhale and the connection you make with the earth as you exhale.

You can add to this sequence by including leg movements. Try rising onto your toes as you breathe in, with heels down gently, bending the knees as you breathe out.

   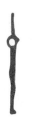 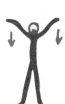

24 October

A physiotherapist friend advises that we should think of the ability to balance like a muscle, and like any muscle, if you want to keep it strong or improve its performance, you have to exercise it regularly. As children, we regularly work our balance muscle when we play, but maybe not so much as we get older. If you feel up to it today, how about having a go at hopping on one foot, then the other, then from foot to foot, exercising your moving balance muscle. Time how long you can stand on one leg before swapping, exercising your static balance muscle. Such timing helps to mark your progress. Or maybe try some balance games you enjoyed as a child, such as hopscotch.

---

25 October

Ever slept funny and woken up with a stiff neck? Or perhaps your neck is stiff from sitting too long at your computer. Try rubbing the rims of your ears with your first finger and thumb. Sounds weird, I know, but it really does help to release the tightness. You do have to keep doing it though at regular intervals throughout the day.

---

26 October

Being aware of our senses and their corresponding elements (smell/earth, taste/ water, vision/fire, hearing/wind or air, touch/atmosphere or ether) is another way we can listen to our inner wisdom. Is there an element we are struggling to connect with? In autumn, for example, you might find it harder to connect with the earth. You may also notice you are feeling lightheaded or a bit scattered. Maybe it's a windy day, which will make it more difficult to feel the earth, to feel grounded. Ask your body what it needs, possibly eating some warm nourishing food such as root veggie soups or stews. Make sure you are warm, and your head isn't getting cold in the wind, and perhaps practise your physical balance. Keep asking and, more importantly, listening and responding to what your body is telling you – this way you can take practical steps to keep yourself in balance and good health.

27 October

Today, I have a variation of the "crocodile posture", which I have always found calming, relaxing and releasing for my lower back and hip area.

Start in the original posture (see 12 May), lying on your front, resting your head on folded arms. Walk your feet and legs out as far as is comfortable, then bend the knees, bringing the lower legs into the air. Allow the lower legs to drop inwards, so one crosses over the other. As soon as they come together, let them bounce back out. If your legs are far enough apart, they will then just flop in again and bounce back out. You can get quite a nice rhythm going here, so that the legs are moving with the momentum and the back and hips can relax. Alternate which leg is in front each time they flop inwards. I like to do this for at least a couple of minutes before coming to a stop, resting for a few breaths in the original "crocodile posture" with heels in, toes pointing out, before releasing and pushing up into sitting.

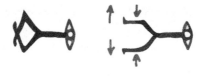

---

28 October

Take a moment to be still, listening to the sound of your breathing. Once it's settled and you are used to the noise, allow yourself to go a little deeper. Can you hear the sound "so" as you inhale? Listen again. Can you hear "ham" as you exhale? Stay with these sounds, expanding with the in-breath, relaxing with the out-breath. Stillness within. Stillness surrounding you.

I love this breath awareness. It helps me to dive into the well of stillness that eternally resides within, whilst consciously changing the energy of my surrounding environment, making a tangible difference.

29 October

One of my favourite postures to open my chest area and help me to breathe more easily is the "chest expansion" – it does what it says on the tin! This is a strong forward bend, so avoid if you have high or low blood pressure, glaucoma, or herniated spinal discs. Go steady if you have back or neck problems.

- Stand with your feet a good hip-width apart, with knees soft – don't lock them out.
- Inhale, raising your arms out to the sides at shoulder-height.
- Exhale, bending your elbows, so you bring your hands towards your collarbones.
- Inhale, stretching your arms forwards. With palms facing away, swoop them down and behind you so that you interlace your fingers behind your back. Feel the lift in your sternum.
- Exhale and fold forwards with lightly bent knees, taking the arms up and back. Let your neck relax, focusing on space between the vertebrae from the tailbone to the crown.
- Pause here, breathing naturally, allowing the arms to move towards the head without forcing them. Feel this move expanding across your collarbone area, rather than nipping the shoulders together. Focus on breathing into the back of your body. We tend to just think about the lungs being at the front of the body, but let the breath move to the back too.
- To come out, lower your arms and release the fingers, bend your knees deeply and push up into standing. You might want to stretch up afterwards.

I like to do this posture three times, holding for a couple of breaths in the forward bend. On the final round, come up and – if you can come into standing without adjusting clothes or stretching up – observe how you feel. Be particularly aware of the chest and underarm – you might detect the subtle expansion of the breath in your ribcage.

30 October

If you are an early riser, you need no telling that the time just before dawn feels very special. Still and quiet, full of promise for the day ahead. It's no surprise that this pre-dawn (90 minutes before dawn) time is considered auspicious by many ancient traditions. It's the perfect time for a peaceful meditation before the busyness of the day, leaving you filled with the creative and vibrant energy of this special time. Each season offers its own dawn gift. Connect with the stillness of winter, the rising creative energy of spring, the coolness of summer and the slowing down and restraint of autumn. Maybe you are able to rise a little earlier each day this week, feeling the energy for yourself.

---

31 October

Time for a confession...I don't much care for Halloween! If it's your thing then I hope you have a fabulous time, with spine-tingling fun and japes. If it's not your thing, then why not spend some time focusing on the light? This could be a walk outside in the daylight, or some quiet time by soothing candlelight. Add an extra layer to this celebration of light by thinking about your ancestors, and if it's not too raw and painful, loved ones who have passed. Give gratitude for their lives, for them being in your life, and for all they taught or gave you. You might want to jot down any notes or flashes of inspiration in your journal. All of these people have helped shape the person you are today.

November

1 November

As the last of the autumn leaves fall, we are encouraged to let go of grief and sadness, whilst giving a last push to release those habits and thought patterns we've been working on through the season. A clear-out of the metaphorical cupboards of your soul if you will. November is a month to bring in more stillness, to find some peace of mind and body, and to consider a future you want to create, the focus of many of our tips this month. Today though, I invite you to slow down. We are getting busier and busier. Consciously slowing down, taking stock of the influences we are allowing into our life and not wandering mindlessly into more busyness, is a useful discipline to cultivate.

2 November

My back absolutely loves this simple exercise:

Lie on your back, with knees bent and feet flat to the floor. As you breathe in, bring your knees into your chest, hugging them as close as you comfortably can, at the same time lifting your head from the floor towards your knees, so you are tucking yourself into a rounded seed-like shape. Release as you breathe out, lowering your head to the floor, then release your knees so you can place the feet on the floor, keeping the knees bent. Repeat this simple exercise at least 10 times before stretching out along the floor for a couple of breaths.

3 November

There's a lot of change in autumn. If I find myself feeling lost, I affirm to myself, "I have all the strength I need, physical and emotional, to move forwards through the ebbs and flows of life, navigating, with ease and joy, whatever change comes my way". This is an affirmation made up of various elements that have felt helpful to me over the years. I hope it helps you too.

---

4 November

Try this methodical way of waking up your body – it is a great way to help you feel grounded and connected to the earth, as well as helping to keep your bones strong and healthy.

Starting at your toes and working your way systematically up your body, lightly tap each one of your bones (keep your focus on the bones, not the muscles). Take your time, feel each bone…each toe, all the bones of the feet and ankles, up the shins, around the knees, the thighs, around your pelvis, gently up your spine, around your ribcage, the collarbones, the shoulder girdle moving down each arm, to the wrists, hands and each one of your fingers. Delicately up the back of your neck, over each part of the skull, tracing the shape of the bones over your face, remembering behind your ears. Be aware of the different sounds each bone makes. How does each bone feel? Do the left and right sound or feel the same?

When you've covered all your body, give yourself a shake out and take a moment to be still. How does your body feel now? I bet you feel alive and tingling all over!

---

5 November

When it's cold or windy outside, make sure you keep your head warm. A simple tip, but honestly, it makes a difference. The cold can aggravate your vata dosha, as does the wind whirling round your head, making you more susceptible to cold and chills, or feeling lightheaded. Personally, I need no excuse to don a hat!

6 November

You know that sensation of weariness when you come in from a busy day, where you feel both wired and tired? This is when we need something to shake off those tension-inducing emotions and move us into our relaxation response. Try any or all of these, though this order works well to help you bring balance to the left and right hemispheres of the brain.

- Give your body a good shake out, every part, to start the release of the stress hormones (see 8 January).
- Do some cross-pattern movements to help you move into the right side of your brain – your relaxation side (see 6 September).
- Lie on your back with your knees into the chest. Clasping around your shins, rock from side to side. Start with minimal movement, gradually increasing the range of the roll, becoming more dynamic each time, working right down to your wrists if you can.
- This one is a bit more dynamic, so only do it if you have no problems with your back, neck or eyes and your blood pressure is normal. You might need to put a blanket down for extra padding. Sit up with your legs crossed (with plenty of space behind you) and hold onto your feet. Keeping hold of your feet, see if you can roll back onto the blanket, with control. You might like to stretch your legs out towards your head, keeping hold of your feet for an extra challenge! Then roll yourself back up into sitting. Repeat a couple of times if it feels right for you.
- Stretch out along the floor, taking a few deeper breaths, making the out-breath longer than the in-breath if you can. Consciously let go of tension and tiredness with each out-breath.
- From sitting, practise a few rounds of alternate nostril breathing (see 14 May).

Now return to your day or evening with calm and clarity.

7 November

Here's an interesting breathing exercise, said to strengthen the lungs against colds, chest infections and the like. As someone who has previously come down with every cold and winter chesty bug going, and with lungs that like a little more support, pretty much every winter used to find me retreating to my bed for at least a week, but a few years ago I thought I'd try this exercise...and I have been pleasantly surprised by its deeply nurturing benefits.

A little word of caution though, this is not a breathing technique for you if you have high blood pressure, heart problems, glaucoma, a detached retina, cataract and/or weak eye capillaries. Far better to stay with some gentle abdominal breathing with no holding of the breath, visualising each breath supporting your lungs.

Practise from sitting or lying down and choose the speed of the count:

- Inhale for a count of six, exhale for a count of six. Repeat this five times.
- Inhale for a count of six, pause (and it is a rest not a forced hold) for three, exhale for six, pause for three. Repeat this five times.
- Inhale for six, exhale for nine. Repeat this five times.

Always treat these breathing techniques with respect. It should always feel relaxed, never forced. If you feel lightheaded or uncomfortable, then stop.

---

8 November

Yesterday, I shared a breathing technique to support your lungs. It also has other benefits you might want to explore. In yoga, the area around the navel is considered a powerful centre for activating your inner strength, creating a calm, clear mind so you can move forwards in life with confidence. Next time you need to find clarity, make decisions that best serve you or connect to your personal power, work the breathing technique I shared yesterday. Here's a reminder along with some added extras!

- Start with a few relaxed breaths (see 5 January), becoming aware of the movement of your navel as you breathe – the area expanding slightly with the in-breath, drawing in towards the spine as you breathe out.

- If it is OK and you are comfortable and happy with breath counting, practise the breathing exercise again with a focus on self-empowerment. Try five breaths of each of these ratios if you can (the same contraindications apply as yesterday).
  - In for six, out for six. This will bring you into the present moment.
  - In for six, pause for three, out for six, pause for three. This brings vitality.
  - In for six, out for nine. Gently firm your abdomen as you breathe to enhance the steadying, grounding properties of the breath. It's also relaxing.

---

9 November

As we've been discovering, autumn gives us the opportunity to let go of what we no longer need. It is also an opportunity to become clear about our purpose or direction in life. Eastern philosophy directs us to our brow chakra, "ajna", to help us gain clarity and become motivated about the future we want. Here are some ideas to help you tap into the wisdom of this chakra.

- Practise listening to your intuition – and it does take practise. Keep listening and trusting your inner voice – the one that comes from your heart or your gut.
- Dreams can be a way our soul talks to us. When you wake up in the morning, lie still for a few moments and see if you can remember any of your dreams. Have your journal handy to make notes. Even if they don't make sense at the time, these whisperings might offer insights at a later date.
- Consider your long-term goals. Do your head and heart tally? Is it your ego talking or are you tapping into your heart's desire? Only you know the answer!
- Wear indigo blue to connect with ajna, or visualise this rich colour flowing across the forehead, soothing the brow and settling the thoughts.
- The beautiful gemstone Lapis Lazuli is the gem to work with to bring balance to the brow chakra.
- If it's OK for you to do, add a drop of relaxing frankincense essential oil to your bathwater or body cream.

10 November

Still a busy mind and find clarity with this short concentration practice. Sit quietly and focus on a spot in the distance for a couple of seconds. Now focus on the tip of your nose, again, just for a couple of seconds. Finally, allow your eyes to rest on the space between your eyebrows, only for a couple of seconds, without straining your eyes. Now relax your eyes, allowing them to gently close. Be still and watch the thoughts that arise. Hopefully this practice has brought some space between the chatter, noting any interesting thoughts that might offer clues as to the direction your soul would like you to follow. Often when we clear the mind chatter, it allows the true, insightful thoughts a chance to be noticed.

11 November

Grounding is a recurring theme throughout autumn. Today, I have a slightly different idea to help you stay centred and connected with the earth. I like to use the essential oil, vetivert. Extracted from the root of a leafy green Indian plant, it smells wonderfully earthy, aromatic, almost smoky. In India, it's known as the oil of tranquillity, which tells you a lot about what it's used for! It keeps us calm under pressure and helps us to deal better with stress. Its grounding and relaxing properties make it perfect for use during times of shock, trauma and separation, helping us to let go without the emotional upset. Try a little spot of the oil at the very base of your spine whenever you are feeling in the clouds or overwhelmed by events. I also find this useful if I've been in the air or on water and still feel like I am, even though I'm firmly on terra firma! A spot of vetivert brings me right back into my body. It's also lovely in an oil burner for a soothing aroma to fill your environment.

As always, check contraindications before using essential oils.

12 November

Here's a quick fix if you find yourself feeling scattered or a bit lightheaded – a simple hand gesture to help you feel centred and grounded again. Bring your hands towards each other with the palms facing the earth. The tips of the thumbs come together and the tips of the index fingers touch, so that you are forming the shape of a triangle, the other fingers spread a little. Hold this triangle, still with the palms facing the earth. For grounding purposes, this is best done if you are sitting or kneeling on the floor. If you can, let your hands connect with the earth and bring your head as close to your hands as you comfortably can, you may even be able to rest your head on the triangle. If you are sat in a chair, let your hands rest on the thighs or a table, allowing your head to relax forwards. Let yourself be still here, feel the connection you make with the earth as you settle, before **slowly** raising the head and releasing.

---

13 November

If you feel adventurous, try a moving balance today. Hold onto something if this is a challenge.

Start by stepping out from one side to the other, getting into an easy rhythm. Next, step out to the right, stepping the left foot behind the right leg, resting on the toes of the left foot. Swap from side to side. Now see if you can put a little hop in as you move from foot to foot. If you are feeling dynamic and are up for a challenge, try keeping the back foot off the floor as you hop from side to side, using your arms to steady you, as if you were skating on ice.

---

14 November

Please be mindful of what you watch or read - there is so much negativity in the world that it's easy to get lost in it all. It makes sense that watching or reading negative, pessimistic or violent content is not going to lead to a calm mind. You may find it more uplifting to focus on love, laughter and learning. Perhaps go further and write more than you read, and create more than you watch.

---

15 November

I know November's full moon as a "frost moon", heralding the colder, frostier weather, reminding us to make our final preparations for winter. Focus on relaxing and reducing, making life as simple as possible for the upcoming season of hibernation. Others will know this moon as the "ancestor moon". In years gone by, we were more reliant on our friends, family and neighbours, particularly during the winter when we might be in need of extra food, shelter or warmth. This was a time to celebrate our relationships and strengthen connections. You might want to continue this tradition, it's a lovely thing to do! Send a special thank you card or gift, or enjoy a celebratory harvest meal or gathering with those you care about.

You may like to extend this further to your ancestors, considering and giving gratitude for all they gave that has brought you to this point. It's also the perfect time to honour anyone close that you've lost, writing a letter of thanks, or noting in your journal all that you loved about them.

---

16 November

Strength comes from having stable foundations. Today, cultivate courage with this simple meditation, connecting with the earth from the Dru Yoga book by Mansukh Pater, Rita Goswami, Chris Barrington, Savitri MacCuish and Louise Rowan, *The Dance Between Joy and Pain*.

- Sit comfortably (on a chair or on the earth). Let your breath settle.
- Take your awareness to the base of your spine and the connection you make with the earth with your legs, feet and sitting bones. Imagine you are rooted to the earth, part of the earth, with no separation.
- Take time to consider the qualities you might associate with the earth – strength, stability, security.
- Each time you inhale, draw these qualities into your legs and sitting bones. As you exhale, let go of tension and anxiety – breathe it out into the earth.

- Now use your in-breath to draw strength and stability into your abdomen, still letting go of tension and anxiety into the earth.
- Repeat, this time drawing the earth qualities into your heart. Rest here, feeling the gentle rise and fall of the sternum. Your body feels strong and stable, your mind calm and peaceful. Affirm to yourself that you are strong and confident.
- Come out of the meditation slowly when you are ready.

17 November

When we start a meditation practice, it can be a challenge to stop fidgeting, particularly with the hands. We can just sit through the fidgeting, letting it run its course, but it can become distracting. Sometimes it's worth making a concerted effort to still our body, with the hands making a good starting point. Try this nifty little trick to help you build steadiness of posture. Place a grain of long-grain rice length ways between your finger and thumb (one in each hand). Now settle into your meditation position, seeing if you can hold your body steady, keeping hold of the grains of rice. If you start to nod off or fidget, you'll drop the rice, so stay focused on keeping the hands still. Eventually, the mind will follow suit and also become more still.

18 November

A while back, I tore the ligaments in my ankle falling down a rabbit hole (very *Alice in Wonderland!*). I was so grateful for my strong and flexible ankles, which recovered relatively quickly. One of the moves I did to help get my ankles back in tip-top workable shape was this...

Very simply, I would describe the alphabet (both upper and lowercase) with my foot. This moves the ankle in all its different ways, bringing strength and flexibility to the foot and the ankle. It also has the advantage of improving our ability to balance. Practise this whenever you think about it, don't wait for an injury!

19 November

When we are anxious, we tend to tense the abdomen, a defence mechanism against an anticipated attack. This tightening can cause pain, bloating and IBS symptoms. Try these three moves to help relax your abdomen. In each move, consciously ask your digestive organs to soften.

- Start by lying on your back with a folded blanket (a heavy wool one is perfect for this) placed over your tummy. Allow your breath to deepen and lengthen, the weight of the blanket providing a feeling of comfort that will encourage your abdominal muscles to release their grip.
- Move into gentle lying twists. Rest for a few breaths at each side (see 5 June).
- Come up into standing to practise a side-stretch. Let your arms slide down one leg, then down the other. If you can, now do a side-stretch with your arms overhead, fingers interlaced. Allow the ribs to move away from the hips as you create space in the abdominal region.

---

20 November

Autumn and winter are times when we might be more interested in how best to support our immune system. One thing you might not have considered is the role our pancreas and adrenals play in our immunity.

The pancreas regulates blood sugar levels after eating. Sugar is widely thought to suppress our immune response, whilst raising inflammatory markers. It can also negatively affect another gland, the adrenals, responsible for how we handle stress, and stress is another factor that can suppress our immunity – it's a double whammy! Today, be curious about the food and drink you consume. Could you reduce your sugar intake? If you are eating sugar, at least try to eat it when you are relaxed and make sure you enjoy it. If, like me, you turn to sugary treats to help you manage stress, this might be something you want to explore, and/or look for alternative ways to manage stress or reduce it.

21 November

In our world of modern technology, this might not be the easiest tip to follow, but I believe you will feel the benefit if you give it a try. How do you feel about reducing or giving yourself a break from all your electronic devices? Yes, that's your phone, tablet, laptop...all of them! Here are a couple of ideas to help you.

- After 30 minutes at a screen, get up and move. Stretch your legs, rest your eyes.
- Make mealtimes a phone-free zone.
- Get into the habit of turning your phone off or switching it to flight mode when not in use.
- Set a period in each day when you switch everything off. It's even better if you can switch off for a whole day every week – believe me, the more you do it the more you'll want to do it, and it gets easier to switch off every time.

---

22 November

Feel strong and grounded with this "warrior posture" flow. If standing is a challenge, sit on the corner of a chair so you can still stretch out your legs (see 25 September for the "seated warrior").

- Walk your feet out into a comfortable wide stance. Turn your right foot out to the right, pushing your left heel out.
- Feel the strength in your legs. Take time to let your breath settle. Lengthen your spine, as if you are putting space at the back of your waist, with shoulders relaxed. Inhale and raise your arms out to the side at shoulder-height, with palms facing down.
- Exhale as you bend your right knee, so the knee sits over the ankle, shin on the vertical. Keep your body tall, your back foot firmly anchored into the earth. Turn to look along your right arm. You can flow in and out of this. Inhale as you straighten your legs, then exhale. Relax your arms. Inhale and lift your arms again. Exhale as you bend the right knee. You might get to a point where you want to pause in the posture, breathing naturally as you hold.
- From this position, allow your left arm to lower down so it rests by the left leg. Raise your right arm up towards your head, softening the elbow.

Inhale, lengthening your spine, and as you exhale, let yourself gently stretch through your right side so you soften backwards towards your left leg, without straightening your right leg.

- Bring yourself back to the centre, with arms out at shoulder-height.
- Exhale, this time lowering your right hand in front of the right knee and, if it feels OK, the left arm straight up. Feel the stretch down the left side now, before returning to the central position.
- Lower your arms and straighten your legs to come out. Walk your legs back to the centre, rest here. When you are ready, repeat the moves to the left.
- When you've finished, give yourself a little shake out and feel the strength in your body.

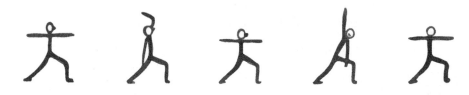

23 November

Settle yourself down in the usual way for today's relaxation, as we transport ourselves to a special place, a place where we can relax and be soothed.

Visualise yourself in your relaxation pose, somewhere outside where you feel you can relax. This can be real or imagined, anywhere you want, so long as you feel safe and able to relax. Perhaps you'll find yourself on a beach, in a wood, in a meadow, at the top of a mountain, or near a river or waterfall.

Can you feel the earth beneath you? What texture are you resting on? Is the earth soft and yielding or firm and supportive? Are you aware of the atmosphere around you? Is it warm or cool?

What sounds are in your special place? Turn your attention to the aromas, breathe them in. Can you taste the atmosphere on your lips? Describe and visualise these to yourself as richly as you can.

Wherever you have chosen to be, give yourself full permission to relax here, healing and rejuvenating, immersed as fully as you can be in the scents, sounds, feel and taste of your special place. When you are ready to return to your everyday world, become aware of your physical body, taking a couple of deeper breaths. Stretch into your fingers and hands, feet and toes. Release your back and neck however you need to, before rolling over and coming into sitting. As you let go of the memory of your special place, know that you can go back there anytime you need to.

---

24 November   Zzz

We know how important it is to get a good night's sleep, but it's not always that easy to nod off, is it?! As a child I found hot milky drinks a comforting bedtime treat and still find comfort in them today. Here are a couple of variations on a theme for kids of any age.

Warm a mug of your milk of choice, drink it as it is or add in one of these:

- A little cinnamon.
- A pinch of nutmeg or turmeric.
- A couple of cardamom pods.
- A chopped-up date (stir in whilst the milk is warming for a sweet chewy treat – this is my favourite!).

---

25 November

Let's get our joints moving and oiled with some circular and swinging movements – they may well click as you start to move, but this should subside the more you do.

- From standing, come onto the toes of one foot and circle the ankle one way then the other, keeping the toes on the floor. Swap feet.
- Now circle your hips in one direction. Start small, with each circle increasing if it feels comfortable. Now back the other way, starting from the smallest circle.
- Stand with your hand resting on a chair (or similar) for balance, swinging one leg forwards and backwards (keep your toes up so you don't scuff them

on the floor). As your hip relaxes into the move you might find you have a greater range of movement. Repeat with the other leg.

- Outstretch your arms in front of you. Circle your wrists one way and then the other.
- Starting with your arms relaxed by your sides, move them in wide circles, forwards and up, behind and down. Now repeat by circling them behind and up, forwards and down.
- Open your arms out wide, at shoulder-height. Bring them in, bending your elbows, so that you can touch your upper arms. Open them out wide and cross again at the elbow, alternating which arm is on top.

Finish by giving your limbs a little shake out. Hopefully you feel warm and energised, and your joints feel looser.

---

26 November

One of the most popular breathing techniques I teach (popular because people find it so effective) is Dru Yoga's "freedom from fear" breath…and it really does do what it says on the tin! You can find it in *The Dance Between Joy and Pain* book.

- Sit comfortably. Shoulders, neck and jaw relaxed.
- Fold your tongue back. Rest the underside of the tongue against the roof of your mouth.
- Hold this, breathing naturally and softly, sounding like someone who is in a deep sleep. Practise for up to five minutes.

Try adding the affirmation, "I breathe out fear, I breathe in peace" with the corresponding breath.

We hold a lot of tension in our mouth. This technique is a clever little hack for activating your parasympathetic nervous system – aka, your relaxation response – bringing calm.

27 November

We've explored a couple of different lying twists during the year. Here is another one I find particularly useful for easing hip and lower back tightness, soothing jangled nerves and aiding digestion. This is not a posture for you if you have acute back problems, sciatica or disc problems, or if you've had recent abdominal surgery.

- Lie on your back with your knees bent and arms outstretched along the floor at shoulder-height. Keeping the knees bent, lightly cross your right leg over your left leg.
- With an exhalation, keeping your legs in this crossed position, allow your knees to relax over to the left. They might not go very far, which is fine – the important thing is that you feel comfortable.
- Bring them back up with the inhalation. Repeat this, rolling the knees to the left at least three more times. Notice if you start to relax into the twist a little bit further each time. On your final round, hold if you feel comfortable, breathing naturally, relaxing the hips, the sides of the torso and across the shoulders.
- Come back up to the centre. Release your legs, stretching out if you need to, before repeating with the left leg lightly crossed over the right (both knees bent) and rolling to your right side.
- Finish by hugging the knees into your chest, gently rocking from side to side, before coming up slowly into sitting.

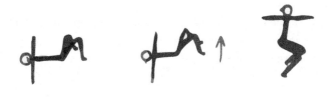

---

28 November

Tired, sore muscles? Try a long soak in a bath of Epsom salts. Lie back and let your aching muscles relax as your body absorbs the magic components. Magnesium sulphate is said to alleviate muscle soreness, although in fairness it could just be the warm water! Either way, it feels nurturing. A 20-minute soak should be plenty. Massage in some body cream or oil before settling down for a good night's sleep, giving your muscle tissue a chance to heal and rebuild.

A word of caution – Epsom salts are not for you if you have high blood pressure, circulatory problems or a heart or kidney condition.

---

29 November

I spoke earlier in the month about being mindful about what you watch and read. The people we mix with can also make a huge difference to our view of life. Look to surround yourself with positive people who share your values. Join groups or connect with people who will help you grow, learn and move forwards. Choose to be with people who support you, maybe even challenge you a little, always in a non-judgemental, no pressure way. Even better if you can commit to connecting with this group or person for a weekly share, as both parties will benefit from being upheld by an honest and supporting friend.

---

30 November

Take your cue from nature and hunker down as the nights draw in. Wrap up warm (getting cold saps vital energy), settling down for earlier nights and stay in bed a bit later. If you can, sleep a little longer. In other words, prepare for a mini hibernation each night – your body will thank you for the rejuvenation time, as we slow down, preparing for the stillness of winter.

December

1 December

Winter. Cold, damp, dark and heavy. There's plenty to look forward to as well, though! The long nights are the perfect opportunity to rest and rejuvenate, time to heal, slowly building energy as we await the return of spring. December also brings lots of festivals of light and celebrations.

To best enjoy all the fun of the season, **balance** is key. Look at your schedule for the month. Where you have late party nights can you pencil in early nights either side, to catch up on sleep? Do you have enough opportunity to get out in the light and the fresh air, to exercise or to just chill out on your own?

When it comes to food, a personal trainer shared with me her way of keeping her food choices balanced during the festivities. If we eat three meals a day, that's 93 meals in December. How many of these are going to be part of celebrations? Let's go for full-on party time and say five a week, giving us 20 indulgent meals over December. That still leaves us with 73 meals where we can make food choices that nourish and support us.

---

2 December

Here is an interesting quote from the ancient sage, Patanjali: "When disturbed by negative thoughts, opposite ones should be thought of."

Our mind has a tendency towards laziness, with thoughts becoming habits. Imagine an index card box, filled with cards. On each card is a thought. Rather than making an effort when thinking, the mind will select one of the cards that's handy at the front of the box (regardless of whether it is true in this moment), instead of taking the time to select a new thought or one that represents the truth. This habitual picking of the same thought creates thought-pattern grooves, if you like. We need to exercise self-discipline, be free thinking in each moment, creating new, more positive grooves. I appreciate this is easier to write than do! Though we can at least have an awareness of another way, and if we don't like how a thought makes us feel, make a conscious resolution to think of something more favourable. It takes practice, consistency and a recognition that we are human, and will make mistakes, which is no problem – we can reset and start again.

---

3 December

Sometimes, we need to stoke our internal fires in winter. Try the "surya" mudra ("surya" means "sun") to bring a little heat to your body. I find it useful for warming me up, helping to fight off colds and shift a sluggish digestive system.

Let your hands rest in your lap, with palms facing uppermost. Fold the ring finger of each hand in towards the palm and hold it in position with the thumb. If you can, rest the thumb on the middle part of the finger, between the finger joints. Stretch out the other fingers.

You can hold this for a few minutes, if you like. Avoid this if you are feeling weak or are excessively underweight.

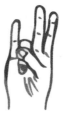

---

4 December

Did you know that electrical devices such as mobile phones, TVs, computers and laptops, along with fluorescent lighting, all contribute to potentially disturbing positive ions in the atmosphere? Positive ions in our environment can, amongst other things, make us feel fatigued, nauseous, lacking in energy, can cause headaches or breathing problems, and affect our ability to concentrate. Negative ions, however, have the reverse effect. If you find yourself feeling jaded during the day, especially if you are working with computers, some simple tweaks to your environment can help.

- At the end of your screen time, spend time outside in nature.
- Have some plants in your work area to purify the air. These breathe in carbon dioxide and breathe out oxygen and negative ions, cleaning up pollutants from the atmosphere. According to a clean air study by NASA, rubber plants, weeping figs and ivy are among the best.
- I like a rose quartz crystal by my laptop as this is said to soak up negative energy. Tourmaline is also a good choice.
- Himalayan salt lamps are believed to soak up negative energy, whilst beeswax candles and indoor running water features produce more negative ions.

---

5 December

Your hands and fingers will love you for this easy massage. Slather on some hand cream (I particularly like to use shea butter as it feels doubly nurturing), working into all the joints of your hands and fingers. Gently pull your fingers (don't crack your joints - note the word "gently"). Massage the palms of your hands, remembering to work into the wrist area and the thumb joint. Work the cream into the backs of your hands. Now, using the first finger and thumb of one hand, massage into the areas between the fingers of the other hand, finishing by applying a little pressure to the fleshy area between the first finger and thumb. Do the same to the other hand. Give your hands and wrists a shake out and thank them for all the hard work they do.

---

6 December

The snow and ice are my inspiration for some moves to warm us up today. Let's go skiing!

- With your feet hip-width apart and knees soft, start with a gentle swinging of the arms, up and down, coordinated with a gentle bounce of the knees.
- As you warm up, and assuming your knees and shoulders are happy, make the swing more dynamic and the knee bounce deeper. Allow your arms to swing up and back. As you swing your arms, you'll probably find your body relaxes forwards.
- If you are feeling particularly energetic, add in a little jump as you swing your arms up. Remember to soften your knees, landing lightly and with control!

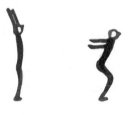

---

7 December

In a world that is increasingly noisy, silence is becoming a rare commodity. Silence is an amazing way of building energy. Few things drain our energy reserves more than constant chatter, or the distraction of external noises such as the TV or radio. Here are a couple of suggestions to help you find peace and build up your reserves.

- Can you dedicate yourself a set period of time for silence (e.g. 15 minutes a day, an hour a week, a full day a month)?
- Set an alarm for every couple of hours. When it beeps, stop what you are doing. For five minutes, just be. Not doing. Not listening to anything. Not watching anything. Just **be**.
- When you wake up in the morning, don't leap straight out of bed, simply lie there, enjoying the peace and silence before the busyness of the day starts.
- Find some silence before you go to bed. Let the chatter die down – you'll sleep better.

Honestly, you'll soon be craving more and more silence – its power is palpable!

8 December

In holistic thinking, the qualities of imagination and intuition are associated with the brow chakra, ajna (see 9 November). If you find yourself in a creative cul-de-sac, try saying the sound "om" to stimulate creativity. I also like to write these letters down, allowing my pencil to play around with the shapes and flow of the letters and, before I know it, I've flowed into another creative expression.

Sometimes our imagination can run wild, which isn't always helpful. This is when I use the sound "mm" (as "mum") to bring calm.

---

9 December

We've practised a few variations – species if you will – of the "cat posture" over the year. This effective and versatile posture can also be practised from a seated position on a chair or, my favourite, sitting cross-legged on the floor.

Sit comfortably with your hands resting on your thighs, with shoulders remaining relaxed throughout. On an out-breath, round your back, drawing the navel in towards your spine, allowing the chin to tuck in a little. Breathe in, lengthening your spine, gently arching in the opposite direction so you are opening your chest, easing the chin up. Repeat as many times as you need to.

You can either stay with this slow, relaxed movement, feeling each vertebra being nurtured, or, if you need to lift your energy and your back is OK, increase the speed a little and the range of movement, so you are gently rocking on your sitting bones. Exaggerate the chest opening and then the rounding, breathing deeply. This variation is also great for stimulating your digestive system.

  OUT IN

10 December

Winter is the time to focus on nurturing comfort food. Swap raw and cold food and drink for warming porridge and hearty stews and soups. Given what we've discussed previously about the immune system (see 20 November), you might also choose to cut down on your sugar and sweet food intake, though a little honey is good as it cuts through mucus. Our digestive fire tends to be a bit stronger in winter, so that we can eat a bit more - the body is so wise, making sure we have all the nutrients we need to see us through the cold months. Eating warm food should make you feel more reassured that you have plenty of food, thereby calming an excessive appetite.

Grains are good in winter, including rice and oats. Barley is particularly useful for drying up dampness within the body. Add warming spices to your cooking too, such as cinnamon, ginger, cardamom and turmeric.

---

11 December

The yoga pose, the "lion", is one of the best when it comes to supporting the mucous membranes, which means it helps to fight off cold bugs. It's also a great posture for opening the carpal tunnel area of the wrists - perfect if you have worked on a keyboard a lot. Plus, it's said to help us stay looking youthful, so it is definitely worth practising! One for doing in the privacy of your own home though, I always think.

- Sit on your heels, with knees apart, big toes together. Adjust this position as necessary. You may want to rest heels or knees on a cushion or sit on a chair and just do the upper body bits.
- Rest the palms of your hands on the floor in front of you (or on a cushion), turning fingers towards you (again, adjust as necessary, you may need to point the fingers away).
- Inhale, as you lift your chin, feeling a nice stretch in the front of your neck.
- As you exhale, stick your tongue out, look to the space between your eyebrows and roar like a lion! Don't hold back!
- Repeat a couple of times.

12 December

Settle yourself down for a beautiful relaxation. You can do this lying down or sitting comfortably. Take a couple of deeper breaths, feeling the heaviness of your body, totally supported by the earth beneath you.

Focus on the base of your spine. Imagine there is a red light, the colour of a ruby. Focus on this ruby light, enhancing a sense of peace and serenity. The red morphs into a glowing orange, like the rising sun. Let this warm orange flow around your lower back and lower abdomen melting away fear, tension and anxiety. Allow your awareness to rise a little, to the level of the navel where you can visualise a strong vibrant yellow. Let the yellow radiate outwards, filling your torso with vitality, strength and creativity. Awareness rises again to the heart centre, visualising emerald green. As this beautiful green fills your chest, be open to love and joy resting in your heart centre. Moving upwards, the green turns to turquoise. Let this soft aqua flow around your neck and throat, gently healing and relaxing. Your awareness rises again, over the face as the blue deepens. On reaching the eyes and the forehead, imagine a rich indigo. Let this deep blue wash over your brow, soothing the mind. Once more, your awareness rises to the crown of the head and above, visualising shades of violet. The violet soon changes to gold. Golden light flows down through the crown of your head, flowing into each part of your body from your crown to your toes – consciously feel it healing, relaxing and rejuvenating every cell of your body. For the last few moments, bathe in this radiant golden light.

When you are ready to come out of the relaxation, take a couple of deeper breaths, wriggle fingers and toes, before stretching and moving your body however it needs to. Roll onto your side to give your body time to come round, before pushing up into sitting.

13 December

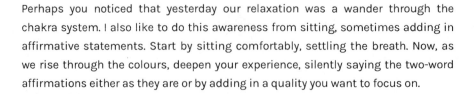

Perhaps you noticed that yesterday our relaxation was a wander through the chakra system. I also like to do this awareness from sitting, sometimes adding in affirmative statements. Start by sitting comfortably, settling the breath. Now, as we rise through the colours, deepen your experience, silently saying the two-word affirmations either as they are or by adding in a quality you want to focus on.

As you focus on the red at the base of your spine – "I am…"
Orange in the lower back and abdomen – "I feel…"
Yellow at the navel – "I do…"
At the heart centre it's green – "I love…"
Turquoise flows around the throat – "I speak…"
Indigo across the brow – "I see…"
As we reach violet at the crown, our affirmation is – "I understand…"

You might want to rest here, focusing on what these statements mean to you – these are good for your journal.

---

14 December

I have another great move for supporting your digestive system. In my experience, it's useful for relieving bloating, whilst also engaging your core postural muscles.

- Lie on your back, with your legs outstretched and arms by your sides.
- Exhale, drawing the flesh in away from your pants, lifting your feet, head and hands (or any combination of these three that feels comfortable for your back – don't strain).
- Be aware not to lift too high. Just lift a few centimetres off the floor.
- Hold for a moment, before relaxing and releasing. You should feel this engaging your abdominal muscles, not straining the back.
- Repeat the move twice more.

15 December

The full moon of December is the "cold moon" – no surprise really as the temperature plummets. By now, we should be ready for the winter months, with all the preparations we've done through autumn. Once again, we are invited to turn within. What do you need to let go of to find stillness? How can you do less? What do you need to rejuvenate? How can you best support your mind and body? All good questions to ask yourself, so that you are ready to move forwards come the spring. Journal, meditate and practise relaxed breathing when this moon is full to help you find clarity. Trust your intuition. Most of all though, stay focused on the light, don't allow negativity to come into your thought process. Stay positive, with no judgement.

Another great way to connect with the energy of this moon, as well as the season, is to get outside and be in the natural world. Feed the birds. Create a natural mandala (see 7 June) using leaves, twigs, stones...whatever takes your fancy. Mindfully lay out your design, enjoying the process and the calm it brings.

---

16 December

If you feel you have a sore throat coming on, try this soothing drink. Steep a couple of fresh sage leaves, or a teaspoon of dried sage, in a mug of hot water, adding a little honey and lemon juice to taste. You can drink this warm or gargle with it once it's cool.

Honey and lemon are classic ingredients for cutting through mucus and easing the sore throat that often accompanies a cold, whilst sage is favoured for its anti-inflammatory and antibacterial properties.

---

17 December

Take a break from your busy day. Be still for a moment. Allow your breath to settle. Let your eyes close if you feel comfortable to do so.

Inhale prana (life force). Feel the prana flowing through your body, nourishing and energising each and every cell. You may find it easier to visualise the prana as light.

Allow yourself to be guided by your inner wisdom. Where in your body needs the extra prana and ultimately your love and attention? Direct the prana to these areas. Let the prana flow and circulate unhindered. Now this is what I call a break!

---

18 December

Today, we practise a movement inspired by the yoga posture, "dancer" – a posture I love, with so many benefits. It's a balance, a gentle back bend and helps us to feel joyful and grounded. For me, though, its real strength is how it helps me to straddle the year – I am rooted in the present moment, leaving the old year behind and moving forwards into the new year with balance and poise.

- From the "mountain pose" (see 9 January), with the left foot firmly anchored, step the right foot back a little way, with the heel off the floor if you can, so you are resting on the toes.
- Swoop your right arm around, resting your right hand on your right thigh. Raise your left hand to your left shoulder, with the palm facing away.
- Inhale, lengthening your spine. Allow your right shoulder to gently roll back, softening the elbow, creating space under the arm. Feel the opening in your chest.
- Exhale, straightening your left arm, pushing your left palm forwards and up a little so it's at eye level. Hold this steady, breathing naturally.
- Release, stepping the right foot back in. Fold into a gentle forward bend to relax your back, before repeating on the other side.

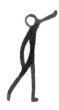

19 December

I know that many people struggle with the lack of daylight during the winter months. It's so important to try to get out into natural light every day if we can, for our fix of sunlight. Even if we don't suffer with full blown Seasonal Affective Disorder (SAD), it is easy to feel fed up with the lack of sun. We want to curl up and hibernate. Our instinct is to comfort eat and sleep, and there is wisdom in this of course, but too much of this can leave us struggling with depleted energy. As always, balance is key.

On a physical level, we do need to experience darkness to activate the pineal gland, which then secretes the hormone, melatonin (known as the "hormone of darkness"), as a response to the dark. This hormone has various therapeutic benefits, and probably many more that we are not yet aware of. Melatonin keeps our circadian rhythms healthy, allowing us to respond to seasonal signals. It's also an important hormone when it comes to helping us sleep (it is interesting to consider how many people struggle with insomnia in our 24-hour culture where the lights are always on and entertainment is available around the clock, meaning no time to be still and embrace the darkness). Dysfunction of the pineal gland has been shown to speed up the ageing process.

Whilst we've thought about getting out in daylight at various points throughout the year, today I encourage you to find harmony with the darkness of the season.

---

20 December

As we head towards the shortest day, it's natural that we mourn the loss of daylight – but wait a minute, don't shy away from the darkness. As we discovered yesterday, it has plenty to offer us. There is a part of our consciousness, linked to our deeper spiritual connection, that will only open in the dark. Taking this a little further, consider how often we hear of people, or you yourself might have experienced, an awakening of our spiritual selves after what is referred to as "the dark night of the soul". We need the balance of light and dark, and the dark is the perfect time to activate the right, intuitive side of the brain.

Alternate nostril breathing (see 14 May) is the perfect practice to embrace the light and dark, bringing balance to every aspect of our being.

Welcome the darkness today, safe in the knowledge that the light is coming soon!

---

21 December

It's the winter solstice today, the shortest day. I find it interesting that there are so many festivals of light around this time of year – the solstice, Hanukkah, Diwali, Christmas – all festivals of hope, reminding us that the light will return. Make time to get outside today, enjoy the sunlight, connecting with the elements. Breathe. Give thanks for the sun and the life-sustaining light it brings. Then cosy up and welcome the darkness, a chance for reflection, for rest and, ultimately, rejuvenation.

---

22 December

Another beautiful practice to do around the shortest day is to take a night-time walk out in nature. A tour around your garden is perfect if you don't feel like going further afield. Make sure you are wrapped up warm and feel safe with wherever you've chosen to stroll. Take a moment for your eyes to become accustomed to the darkness, slowly bringing an awareness of your surroundings. How does the world look in the dark? What do you see that you don't see in the daylight? Being out after dusk helps us to stimulate the part of our brain, linked to intuition and spiritual connection, that only awakens in the darkness, so enjoy this magical experience.

---

23 December

Need a shot of energy? This energising breath always helps me.

Stand or sit in a comfortable position, with the back nice and tall. Raise your arms out to shoulder-height, with elbows bent and palms facing forward. Inhale, bringing the forearms together. Exhale as you open the arms out (I know this might feel counter-intuitive!). Repeat a few times, each in-breath filling the lungs with prana, feeling it expanding in the chest and torso. Feel the opening in the back of your body and into the lower lobes of the lungs. Start with a couple of rounds, don't overdo it. You can steadily build up repetitions over time.

24 December

Holiday season can be a lot of fun. It can also be painful, lonely, stressful, anxiety-inducing and hard work. It's good to acknowledge when we might not be feeling so cheerful, recognising what emotions are coming up for us. Sit with it, journal about it, consider what you can do to honour yourself.

Throughout this book there are tips for soothing and relaxing mind and body, for boosting energy and balancing emotional responses. One thing we haven't touched on though is loneliness, an emotion which, in my experience, can be acutely felt at this time of year. We can be with people and still feel lonely. There are many self-help approaches to loneliness. A quick internet search will yield a host of ideas. Here are a few of the perhaps less obvious ones:

- Light a candle. There is something about this act that connects us to the wider world, reminding us we are not alone.
- Pay particular attention to your own self-care needs – take time to rest, nurture yourself with good food, move your body, indulge in some pampering, be creative.
- Do something that helps or reaches out to someone else. Chances are you are not alone in your loneliness!
- Try this expansive breathing technique. From standing or sitting, bring your hands in front of your heart centre. Inhale (this can be quite a strong breath if it feels OK), taking your arms out wide, opening your chest so you almost feel like you are about to step forwards. (You can actually step forwards with each in-breath if you want to make it stronger, making sure you do an equal number on both sides.) Exhale, bringing your hands back to the centre. Repeat at least five times. Try adding a positive affirmation with each in-breath. When you've completed your rounds, be still for a moment, focusing on the space between your hands, before giving your upper arms a nice reassuring rub and a hug to finish.

If you love the busyness of the holiday season, please look out for those who may not share your enjoyment. Maybe there is something you could do to help ease their loneliness.

25 December

Merry Christmas! I hope you have a fabulous day.

This time of the year is not easy or fabulous for everyone, though. As mentioned yesterday, it's a time that can bring up all kinds of emotions - anxiety, loneliness, irritation, anger, guilt and grief, as well as joy. Please take some time today to honour yourself. If you find yourself feeling overwhelmed or in need of five minutes of peace, take yourself off somewhere quiet (honestly, locked in the bathroom is my quiet space on Christmas Day!) and try this simple breath.

From sitting or standing, bring your arms out in front, at shoulder-height, with palms facing your chest as if you are hugging a tree. Inhale, drawing your palms in towards your chest, feeling your sternum lift, opening your heart centre. Exhale, pushing your palms away, returning to the starting position. Continue with this beautiful flow as many times as you want, as the breath becomes slow and steady. Consciously breathe in calm, love and patience. Draw in whatever you feel you need. As you breathe out, push away the busyness, the anxiety, the irritation, letting go of whatever is unsettling you.

For those who love the day, I also urge you to practise this breath, sending out your love, peace and joy to the world.

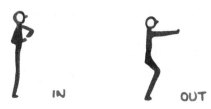

IN   OUT

---

26 December

Overindulgence goes hand in hand with festivities! After a big meal, our digestive system needs extra energy to digest all those festive goodies, but this can leave us feeling sleepy. Instead of a snooze, why not go for a gentle stroll? Nothing too exerting, just a little walk to stoke the digestive fires. This can help you manage your blood sugar levels, burn off a few calories and kick-start the digestive process.

---

27 December

We are well into cold and flu season. Here is another mudra you might want to add to your winter bug first-aid kit! "Linga" (upright) mudra is said to build our resistance to colds, coughs and chest infections – it is particularly helpful for loosening mucus from the lungs. Don't practise it if you have a fever or existing heart or lung conditions.

With your palms together, interlace your fingers. Keeping one thumb upright, allow the index finger and thumb of the other hand to encircle it. Try this a couple of times a day, holding for up to 15 minutes at a time.

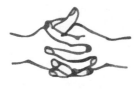

---

28 December

The end of the year is fast-approaching! I hope that as we have flowed through the seasons you have found some amazing health and wellbeing tips that have resonated and supported you. More than anything, though, my wish is that I have inspired you to be proactive when it comes to your wellbeing. Ayurvedic philosophy encourages us to focus 90% on prevention and 10% on cure because, of course, prevention is so much easier than cure! Please, take the best care of yourself, you really do deserve it.

29 December

Over the last 12 months I have given you many wellbeing ideas and practical things you can do at home. The benefits of all these cannot be reaped by just reading about them, though – you need to do them! My tip today is to practise what you've read in this book. Pick out the techniques that have resonated the most, highlighting them for easy access. Dip in and out as suits you. Maybe you will choose to start reading through the book again in the new year – your experience and awareness will be different with every read.

Most of the tips take only a couple of minutes. You deserve this time, and I promise you'll feel the benefit so much more than just reading about them.

---

30 December

The year is nearly over. I hope it has been a good one for you. Today, I will be honouring the year, giving gratitude for all that it has brought. The truth is some years are better than others, but whatever the year has brought, there are always silver linings to be found.

I settle myself down with a cuppa and my notebook, reflecting on the year that has been. What have I enjoyed? What went well? What have I learnt? What about new experiences? What do I not want to repeat next year?! Take time to say thank you.

This is also an opportunity to consider how I would like next year to shape up. I make a note of my wildest dreams (as the song "Happy Talk" from the musical *South Pacific* by Richard Rodgers and Oscar Hammerstein goes, "You got to have a dream. If you don't have a dream, how you gonna have a dream come true?"), as well as my more manageable goals and hopes for the year. You might like to write your ideas down, illustrating this important treasure map of self-discovery. Keep your map handy for the year ahead – let it guide your actions and your thoughts.

31 December

As we head into a shiny new year, with all that it promises, I would like us to remember we are all beautiful beings of light, every one of us. Affirm "I am capable of amazing things" because we all are...YOU are. Wishing you much love and joy for the year ahead.

"I am capable of amazing things."

Printed in Great Britain
by Amazon

28340415R00126